PRAISE FOR KIMBERLY SNYDER AND
THE BEAUTY DETOX FOODS

"I don't like to diet. I like to eat right and that's what Kim's philosophy is all about. Her food program has had such an impact not only on my body but my health in general. She's brilliant."

—Drew Barrymore

"Kimberly Snyder's The Beauty Detox Solution *is a must-read that intelligently highlights the importance of incorporating large amounts of greens and plant foods in our diet. It also provides readers with innovative ways to maximize their consumption."*

—Dr. Mehmet Oz
Host of *The Dr. Oz Show* and co-author of the *You* book series

"I learned about Kimberly and her Glowing Green Smoothie through my husband (Josh Duhamel) who started making it for us. It really is just amazing! It gives me so much energy and makes me feel better about myself and my skin. I can really feel the difference. I also love her food, and feel my best when I am eating it, as it energizes me so much."

—Fergie

"The Beauty Detox Foods is a helpful book. I love all Kimberly's delicious, healthy recipes and treats! She is the originator of my favorite drink ever, the Glowing Green Smoothie, which I drink every morning. Kimberly is also so smart, and her fresh new outlook on nutrition—which stresses lifestyle changes, not fad diets—has been a big awakening for me. I have never felt better since I've been on her program!"

—Hilary Duff

"Ever since I started following Kimberly's advice in her book The Beauty Detox Solution*, my body has never felt better! My stomach is flatter, I have more energy and I find it much easier to maintain my ideal weight. I never, ever miss a morning with her Glowing Green Smoothie; it's made my body crave healthy, green foods. I've always considered myself a very disciplined and healthy eater, but her book really cleared up some of my misconceptions about what foods really are the best choices."*

—Dita Von Teese

"Kimberly has changed the way my whole body works. She has helped my overall health and digestive issues. I feel healthier and have more energy when I perform."

—LeAnn Rimes

"I have learned so much about nutrition from Kimberly. Her recipes taste so great that it's hard to believe you can eat this healthy and yet feel so satisfied and content. Her philosophies and food have really had a tremendous impact in all aspects of my life."

—Ben Stiller

"Kimberly is a game changer! By following her nutritional program, for the first time in my life I'm eating healthy and enjoying it! I always start my day with her Glowing Green Smoothie and my energy has increased and I feel great."

—Channing Tatum

"Experiencing Kimberly's food on set is what made me change the way I viewed living foods. It isn't all nuts and oils! Her food program will appeal to everyone and take away the fear associated with a greens-based diet."

—Olivia Wilde

"I drink Kimberly's Glowing Green Smoothie every day! It really has made a dramatic difference in the way I feel and I have so much more energy. Kimberly's recipes are so tasty, too! I always feel better when I am following her plan and eating her food."

—Josh Duhamel

"I was introduced to Kimberly and her Glowing Green Smoothie and it's now the staple of my daily regimen that I won't skip. When it comes to health and nutrition, Kimberly is a real expert. Her nutritional concepts are easy to follow, make sense and will increase your energy and vitality. After reading this book there really isn't an excuse not to make healthy food with so many amazing and delicious recipes."

—Owen Wilson

"When I am following her plan there is a dramatic difference in the way I feel. I drink her Glowing Green Smoothie every day. She is just a genius in the kitchen, as she is able to create great tasting, healthy recipes so you never feel like you're missing out, which is why her plan has been so effective for me."

—Vince Vaughn

"To say that Kim Snyder changed my life is a total understatement. I went from lethargic to energetic, dull tired skin to glowing skin, I keep weight off effortlessly, my mood is much more stable and I generally enjoy my life at least 50% more. I wake up every morning alert, happy and fulfilled. Meeting Kim and working with her are two of the best things that ever happened to me. I will never go back to a pre-Kim life!!"

—Laura Benanti

"Kim's philosophy turns our conventional thinking about food upside down. Have an open mind! Eating her incredible plant-based recipes, and starting every day with the GGS, there is no more crash and burn. I have sustained energy throughout the day, no more cravings, and know that I can enjoy everything I'm eating without feeling any guilt. It's the end of calorie counting and the beginning of looking and feeling the best you've ever felt."

—Christine Taylor

"Through Kim's help, my skin has become so much clearer and brighter. I have kicked the fatigue and just have much more vitality. To me the key word is lifestyle. It is not a diet, it is making decisions about my health that positively impact my life in every aspect. The Glowing Green Smoothie has been integral for me to maintain energy throughout the day, especially when I'm working long hours on set. I know that the changes Kimberly has made in my diet have led me to feeling the best I have in years."

—Teresa Palmer

"I love Kimberly Snyder so much I want to put her in my pocket and take her everywhere. Apparently that's a little creepy and impossible, but I do get to bring the tools she's empowered me with from her books to every character, act and balance of my life. Her sensible and passionate education of energizing and detoxifying my life gives me this wonderful 80/20 balance that I know I can sustain. It's hard to believe how much energy I have when I'm implementing her program. I just can't get tired. It really works. Try it. You'll like it!"

—Abigail Spencer

"Kimberly's knowledge of nutrition is excellent and her natural foods program produces results."

—Kevin James

"Making Kim's green smoothies in the morning gives me enough energy to fly through the rest of the day. I couldn't imagine a better way to start it off!"

—Malin Akerman

"Kimberly is beyond beautiful. I was able to lose all of my baby weight, and keep it off, by following her program and drinking her Glowing Green Smoothie."

—Jillian Barberie
Former host of Fox morning show *Good Day L.A.*

"Kimberly has changed my view on healthy eating. The impact she has made on my energy level and overall health has been amazing."

—Eddie Cibrian

"Kim Snyder has completely changed my life for the better. My days are long and require a lot of energy and focus. Her program not only has me at a higher level of fitness than I've ever been, but I'm energized and focused all day long. Kimberly and her program will be a part of my life forever. She is a product of what she preaches. She glows."

—Steven Pasquale

"The misuse of the word literally *is one of my more persistent pet peeves so I don't mean this lightly or incorrectly when I say Kimberly's nutritional philosophy and methods have* literally *changed my life. After following her ideology for just a brief amount of time, I found that I possessed an energy I haven't known since I was a kid—an ability to connect and focus that has hugely aided me as an actor. At events I consistently find myself in the middle of a passionate and almost completely unsolicited rant to a stranger about Kimberly's ethos and program. Enjoy!"*

—Justin Long

THE
BEAUTY
DETOX
FOODS

Discover the Top 50 Beauty Foods That Will Transform Your Body and Reveal a More Beautiful You

KIMBERLY SNYDER, C.N.

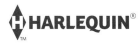

THE BEAUTY DETOX FOODS
ISBN-13: 978-0-373-89264-8

Photos of Fresh Asian Cucumber Spring Rolls, Gluten-Free Vegan Lasagna Supreme, Gluten-Free All-Veggie Pizza, Spiralized Asian Veggie Salad, Portobello Mushroom Burgers and Stuffed Acorn Squash by Zade Rosenthal. Photos on pages 130 and 148 by Josh Maready.

All other photography, including cover shot, by Ylva Erevall.

Image of boat near James Bond Island, page xiv, by John Arnold Images/Masterfile.

The health advice presented in this book is intended only as an informative resource guide to help you make informed decisions; it is not meant to replace the advice of a physician or to serve as a guide to self-treatment. Always seek competent medical help for any health condition or if there is any question about the appropriateness of a procedure or health recommendation.

The Glowing Green Smoothie is a trademark of Kimberly Snyder.

Library of Congress Cataloging-in-Publication Data
Snyder, Kimberly.

   The beauty detox foods : discover the top 50 beauty foods that will transform your body and reveal a more beautiful you / Kimberly Snyder.

      p. cm.
      Includes bibliographical references and index.

   ISBN 978-0-373-89264-8 (pbk.)
   1. Detoxification (Health).   2. Nutrition.   3. Beauty, Personal.   4. Self-care, Health.   I. Title.
   RA784.5S65 2013
   613.2—dc23
   2012017080

www.Harlequin.com

Printed in U.S.A.

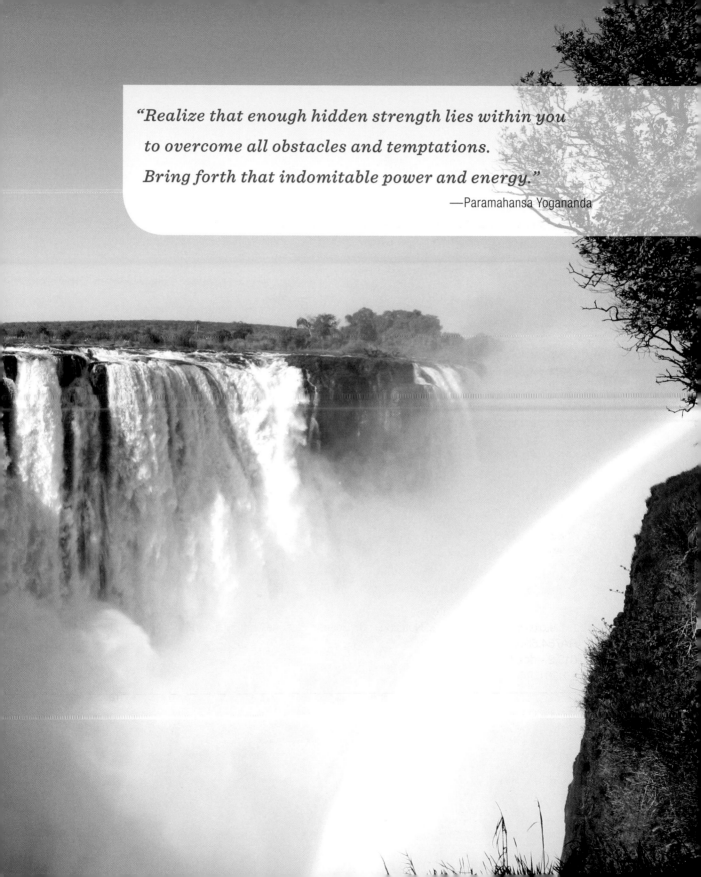

"Realize that enough hidden strength lies within you to overcome all obstacles and temptations. Bring forth that indomitable power and energy."

—Paramahansa Yogananda

CONTENTS

PART II

BEAUTY DETOX FOODS

PART III

BEAUTY DETOX RECIPES

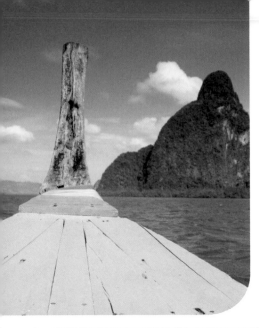
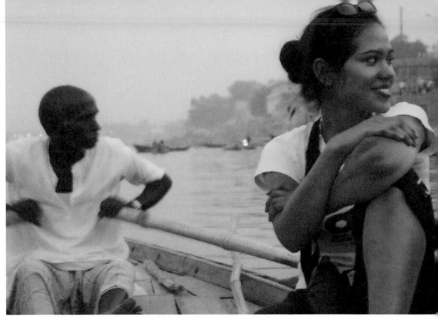
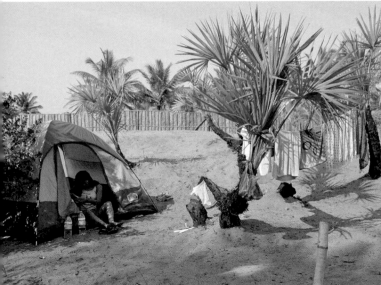
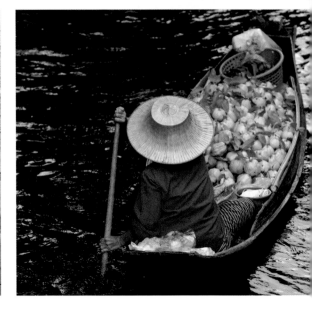
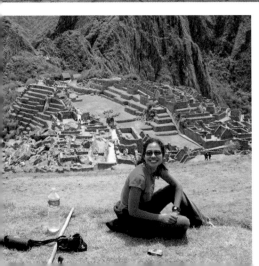
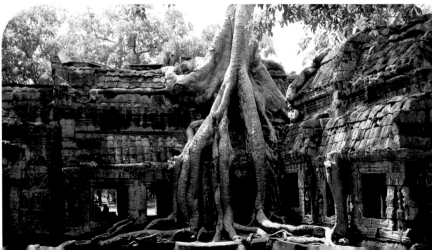

INTRODUCTION

Whether you read my first book, *The Beauty Detox Solution*, are a member of my online community at kimberlysnyder. net or are joining me for the first time, welcome to the journey toward realizing your birthright: ultimate health and beauty. Like most people, I've been through the gamut of beauty issues: flabbiness and excess weight that started in my junior year of college, hair that felt like steel wool and major acne. Now, all are long gone. What happened? First, I tried everything from fat-free to low-carb diets, and I tried recording every calorie in a food journal. I used every hair product you can imagine. I tried prescription acne creams, and even briefly went on antibiotics. Nothing worked for more than a short while.

Then I got a chance to do something pretty extreme: global backpacking. My journey was not of a sheltered, live-in-a-villa-for-a-few-months variety. It was dusty, dirty and (now that I look back at it) somewhat dangerous. I spent the majority of time traveling through Asia and Africa, but also South America, Australia and Eastern and Western Europe. For three years, I had adventures across over fifty countries that could fill a book, but I also got to observe firsthand how health and beauty are seen in the rest of the world.

Contracting viruses and getting seriously ill on two separate occasions in Nepal and India, I ended up under the care of doctors in both countries—and both experiences made me seriously consider different approaches to health care than what we have in the United States. These doctors asked me something no Western doctor had ever brought up. To be blunt, in both cases their first question was about my poop. At first I was confused, then slightly embarrassed, then confused again as to why they were talking about "toxins" rather then just jamming pills at me like the doctors back home. They gave me a suppository and advised me that I would not heal until toxins were forced to exit my body. In India, a common saying is that "Constipation is the mother of all disease." Indians stress the importance of correcting the root cause, while in the United States, we focus on a pill-popping strategy *after* troubles arise, and then spend more money on digestive aids (antacids, laxatives and the like) than on any other over-the-counter medication. Later, I heard the same idea about digestion and constipation, although worded slightly differently, in the Philippines.

I also marveled at the vibrant hair and skin of the women living in countries like Indonesia, Thailand and Malaysia. At the same time, living in those countries for stretches of time forced me to eat many of the native foods they were eating, including papaya and coconut. Gradually, my skin started improving. I also learned about native probiotic-rich foods firsthand, since it would have been unthinkably rude to refuse the *airag* (fermented mare's milk) that was proudly offered to me by three generations of a family whose *ger* (tented home) I camped on the floor of in Mongolia. Don't worry, we have much tastier options for eating cultured, fermented food. But I saw the benefits. In Japan, I marveled at the commonality of porcelain-smooth skin. I used to spend hours wandering around the alleys of traditional markets, looking at all the different types of sea vegetables that are a mainstay of the Japanese diet.

In the end, having immersed myself in native foods and practices, my hair became shiny and thick, my skin became radiant and, in all the years since then, I've never once had to go back to dieting. Not once.

I was so fascinated with what I learned on my travels that, after coming back home, I became a clinical nutritionist, combining the best health and beauty secrets from around the world with subsequent years of study.

My message of becoming attuned to nature to be our most beautiful and healthy selves started to catch on, and I began to work with some of the biggest celebrities in the entertainment world, getting them ready for red-carpet events and upcoming roles for major Hollywood films, as well as concert tours. I create their nutritional plans and often prepare their food on a regular basis, including before and during the production of films. This inspires me to keep developing foods and recipes to suit my clients' tastes, while always adhering to my nutritional philosophy.

I wrote *The Beauty Detox Solution* in 2011 and was inspired to write this second book, *The Beauty Detox Foods,* to focus on the beauty foods found everywhere in nature and to offer more recipes. I also offer a summary of the concepts in *The Beauty Detox Solution,* and discuss additional important topics. You'll be happy to find that most of the foods in this book are at your local farmers' market or neighborhood grocery store. Beauty is right at your doorstep. Looking and feeling beautiful and maintaining a healthy weight are actually simple. Our best beauty weapons are born in nature and are in abundance all around. You only have to eat the right beauty foods in the right way and cleanse on an ongoing basis to look and feel your absolute best.

You are going to be eating an abundance and an array of plant foods, which contain a plentiful supply of complex phytonutrients, including vitamins, minerals, fiber and enzymes that nature creates in perfect ratios. It will feel right to you, as you continue along the path because, deep down, Beauty Detox principles and foods resonate with your intuitive connection with nature. As you go back to your natural way of eating, you'll become more naturally beautiful.

When your cells and blood are clean and detoxified, your body will be able to function optimally and you'll assimilate the full spectrum of minerals in your food. As a result, your skin will become smoother and radiant from within, your eyes will lose their dark circles and puffiness, and your hair will grow in lustrous and thicker.

Following this Beauty Detox program will also free you from the dreaded, never-ending battle with dieting. How much of your life have you spent searching for ever-new ways to diet and lose weight? From cleanses consisting of powdered supplements to dabbling in an Atkinseque carb restriction or a microwaved, processed-foods plan, chances are you've tried a lot. The problem, which we've all discovered, is that each of these new ways to lose weight leaves you feeling deprived and unsatisfied. A major reason that diet foods never work for the long run is that they cut you off from your connection to nature. Diet foods are highly refined, formulaic creations made with ingredients from the lab. With the Beauty Detox program, you'll be eating real food that your grandparents would have recognized. As you start to increase the abundance of these magical, sometimes deceptively humble and common beauty foods, you'll start to decrease your intake of foods that don't serve you anymore. You'll also become naturally addicted to feeling energized, and you'll experience more glowing skin and a shrinking belly. These dramatic results will motivate you to stick with this new way of eating.

In Part I, you will review the essential principles that make up the core of the program. Please don't skip this section! Be sure to read it, even if you have read *The Beauty Detox Solution*. Understanding the concepts in Part I is critical to making this program work for you, especially because the information on this program is different from any other diet or detox book you may read. It is the sum of knowledge I've learned from many different teachers, health institutions and trainings, as well as on my around-the-world journey. The concepts presented here are based on sound, thorough research and the work of many doctors, scientists and research institutions. I have cited numerous studies and specific research throughout for your reference, so that you can see how the science supports the program. Some of the principles have not yet trickled into the mainstream health and nutrition practices, but please keep an open mind as you read, and remember that many tenets of health that are widely accepted now—such as that smoking cigarettes increases your odds of getting lung cancer—were not always mainstream ideas.

Then, in Part II, I discuss the top 50 Beauty Detox foods, organized by common beauty concerns. Part III offers exciting recipes that will increase your Beauty Energy, are easily digestible and incorporate the top beauty foods, to make becoming beautiful fun, delicious and an easy part of your lifestyle.

There is an exhilarating and liberating new path ahead to abundant health and beauty beckoning you to follow it. Just turn the page.

In health, true beauty and love,
Kimberly

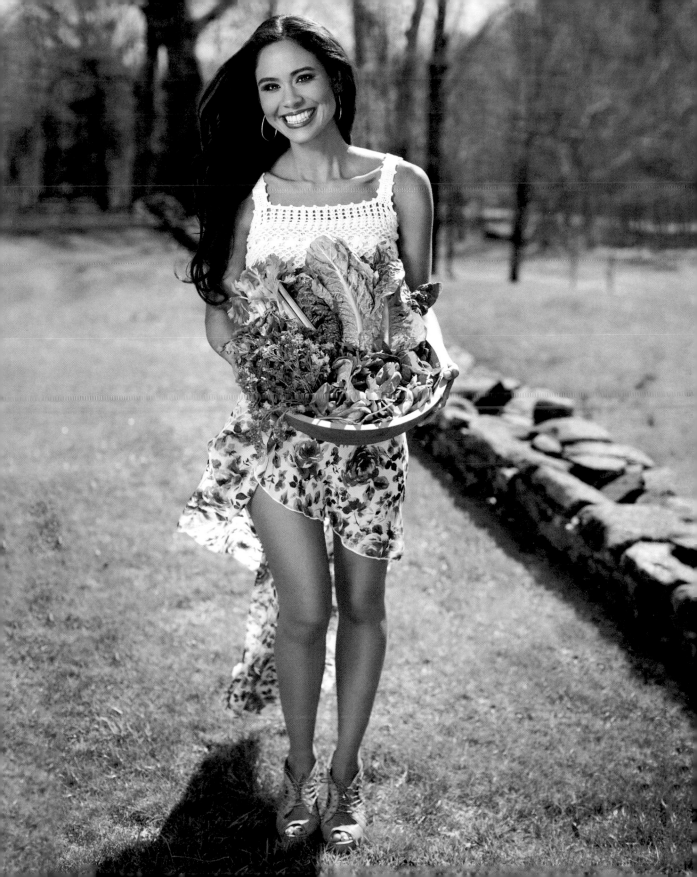

BEAUTY
DETOX
101

The connection between food and beauty is incredibly powerful. Just by changing the foods you eat, you can radically change the way you look and feel.

In the following chapters, you'll get a basic grounding in how to clear out from your body all the junk and toxicity —the clogging sludge that keeps you from looking and feeling your best—and begin to eat truly beautifying foods in a strategic way that will add sheen to your hair, put a sparkle in your eyes, and firm up and tighten your skin.

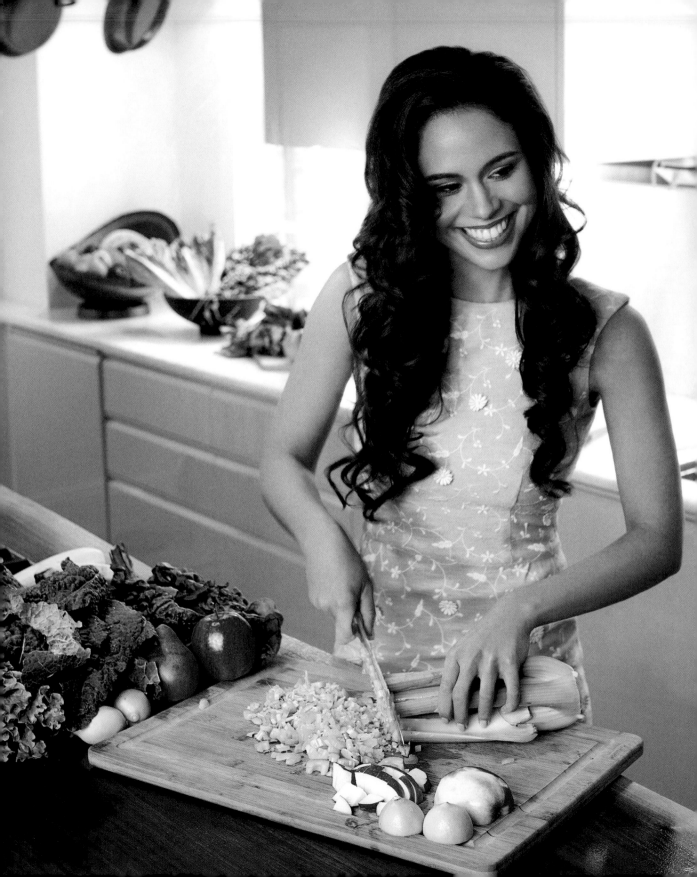

THREE BEAUTY DETOX PRINCIPLES

1

One of the most important assets you have in your quest for beauty is energy. Energy is a key factor in your ability to shed weight easily and permanently, achieve great health and look your most beautiful. Energy regenerates your liver and other tissue cells, flushes toxic waste from the body, helps maintain your ideal weight, keeps your skin's collagen smooth and your hair healthy, and keeps blood from stagnating into dark under-eye circles. The more energy you have, the better you feel and the more beautiful you become.

What eats up energy? The quick answer: digestion. Yes, digestion! Did you know that the full process of digestion takes more energy than any other internal function of the human body? Some experts estimate that digestion takes as much as half or more of your total energy.[1] Digestion is the key that can elevate your beauty to the highest levels or, adversely, take you down, by sucking up precious energy that could be used for other processes. Beauty Detox Foods are designed to free up energy from digestion, which is the single most important way to redirect large amounts of energy to make weight loss easy and help you look your most beautiful.

How Your Face Reveals Inner Health

For over five thousand years in Chinese medicine, practitioners have understood that uneven color and texture, patchiness, lines, breakouts and other issues with your face can be indicative of deeper issues going on within your body and in your organs.[2] Similar to acupuncture, face-mapping is rooted in the belief that all parts of the body are intrinsically connected. It is a complex art, but here are some examples of commonly held ancient Chinese beliefs about what you might learn from examining your face:

○ Breakouts around the chin/jaw area could signal a hormonal imbalance and congestion in the colon.

○ Lines above the upper lip might indicate stagnation or blockages in the digestive tract, specifically relating to the organs of the stomach and small intestines. This can be attributed to the accumulation of acidic waste and toxicity, which is not adequately leaving the body.

○ Deep laugh lines (and the nasolabial line) relate to your lung and liver. These lines could be due to smoking or shallow chest breathing, indicating that not enough oxygen is getting into the lungs (yoga definitely helps with this) or a colon that is so backed up that your lung meridian is being impeded. The lungs and colon are considered yin-yang organs. These laugh lines may also mean you have an overloaded liver.

○ A lined forehead might point to congestion, and specifically a blocked, toxin-filled colon and gallbladder. Among the contributors to this may be consuming a lot of dairy, cooked oils or processed foods. On the other hand, a person might have a good diet but is not cleansing properly or adequately to keep up with the toxicity the good diet is releasing.

○ Dark under-eye circles or puffiness may indicate adrenal exhaustion. Too much caffeine, a lack of sleep or too much stress may cause this.

○ Crow's feet around the eyes may signal that your adrenals are being overtaxed and that your body is overly acidic and imbalanced.

○ Patchy skin or lines high up around the cheekbone area may be associated with heart issues. These could be due to eating too much cholesterol, animal products or cooked oil.

The good news is that your cells regenerate. If you take positive steps now to improve your diet and cleanse your body, you can reverse damage and make major improvements in your overall heath and beauty.

Your body's systems are always trying to maintain perfect balance, which leads to superior health and beauty, but this is possible only after you have cleansed yourself of toxic material that constantly accumulates. The more efficiently you digest food (in other words, the less energy your body has to spend on digesting), the more energy your body has to clean out the old toxic material and perform all those beautifying processes. The toxic sludge amasses at a much faster pace when you're not digesting your food efficiently.

Detoxing yourself by getting rid of old waste is the key to allowing your digestion to function optimally. When you loosen the toxic sludge from your system, your energy will automatically increase because your body will be able to perform digestive and other functions efficiently and with much less effort. Thanks to that renewed energy, you will also lose weight and look years (or even decades) younger. Your skin will radiate and your hair will grow in with vibrant body and a healthy sheen.

Most diets focus on the number of calories or grams of carbs and protein to consume, yet they make no effort to deduce how efficiently—or not—your system can break down or use any given food. These eating plans don't consider Beauty Energy and how it's used up in digesting foods that are difficult to break down. Calories and grams of carbs and proteins alone don't give a holistic picture of how healthy a food is within the human body, how nutrient-dense it is or how much fiber it contains. Nor do they give you any clues as to the amount of foreign chemicals, preservatives and additives that may be in that given food. That is the very reason that dieting and losing weight have always seemed like such a miserable chore and struggle, a struggle that most of us feel we are losing, along with energy levels. And it's one of the reasons people age at such an accelerated rate. There's more to our achieving thriving health and beauty than adding up a bunch of numbers. Don't worry, because you are soon going to learn the easy way to lose weight and get your energy back again.

The high content of mineral-, enzyme- and fiber-rich Beauty Detox Foods will help cleanse and unclog the waste from the intestines so that your body can start to absorb nutrients optimally. But building up toxic waste in the body can take many years, even decades, so detoxification on a deeper level is not something that happens instantly. It should be a gradual, controlled and regulated process . . . and it needs to take place continuously to get the tangible results you are after. In fact, detoxification that happens too quickly can be very uncomfortable—you can feel or actually become ill. But you can start to see changes fairly quickly by making important shifts in the foods you eat.

Overfed, Yet Starving for Beauty Nutrients

One reason people tend to overeat and struggle so much with calorie counting and portion size while still being hungry is that their bodies aren't fully absorbing nutrients. Nutrients are absorbed through tiny hairlike villi along the walls of your intestines. You have over seven thousand feet of surface area in the small intestine.

However, if the tiny villi get clogged, you won't feel nourished, no matter how much you eat. The villi are easily clogged by the waste products of foods that your body can't metabolize and utilize efficiently, and that also promotes the production of excessive mucus or yeast. Just a few examples of these clogging foods are processed foods that contain chemicals or additives, refined sugars, cow's milk and other dairy products, excessive animal protein, and white flour–based foods.

Another way the villi can get clogged is from the excessive growth of yeast and fungus in the body. In his book *The pH Miracle,* Robert Young, Ph.D., explains how yeast and fungus impede nutrient absorption: "They can cover large sections of the membrane lining the inside of the small intestine, displacing probiotics and preventing your body from getting the good stuff out of what you eat. This can leave you starving for vitamins, minerals, and especially protein, regardless of what you actually put in your mouth. I estimate that more than half of adults in the United States are digesting and absorbing less than half of what they eat."[3]

When you aren't absorbing nutrients, your body tells you to keep eating, although you have just been fed. Thus begins the utterly deflating and guilt-inducing cycle you may be all too familiar with: eating more, even when you know you've just eaten plenty of food and, yes, plenty of calories. I totally understand the frustration and have experienced it myself. *Why am I still hungry when I just ate two full plates at the buffet?*

Raw food nutrition pioneer Dr. Norman Walker writes in depth about the effects of eating processed and devitalized foods. As he explains in *Colon Health:* "If a person has eaten processed, fried and overcooked foods, devitalized starches, sugar and excessive amounts of salt, his colon cannot possibly be efficient, even if he should have a bowel movement two to three times a day."[4]

In other words, the prevalence of bowel movements, although very important, does not necessarily indicate how cleansed and toxin-free your body is. You can still have clogged intestinal villi, as well as impaction and waste matter pushed deep into your body, which keeps you from absorbing the nutrients you need.

At its most basic level, Beauty Detox comes down to three simple guidelines:

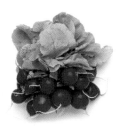

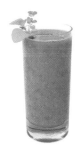

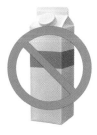

Eat more veggies and fewer animal products

Drink the Glowing Green Smoothie (or Juice) every day

Give up dairy

EAT MORE VEGGIES AND FEWER ANIMAL PRODUCTS

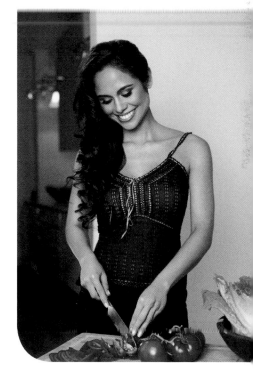

The best thing you can do to improve your overall health and beauty is to fill your diet with whole, unrefined plant foods. As pointed out in *Forks over Knives: The Plant-Based Way to Health*, "Natural, plant-based foods provide all the essential nutrients needed for a well-balanced and healthy diet, as there are no nutrients found in animal-based foods that are not abundantly available in plant foods, with the exception of vitamin B_{12}. And you can supplement vitamin B_{12} for insurance."[5] In the past, B_{12} was obtained in adequate amounts from a plant-based diet, because microorganisms in the soil manufacture B_{12}. But today, foods are sanitized and scrubbed of soil exposure. Although you may choose to keep some meat in your diet for taste, social, familial or any other reasons, there is no nutritional reason to do so. We discuss protein (that inevitable topic when the notion of a plant-based diet is discussed) in the following section, but rest assured that if your diet isn't deficient in calories, it is practically impossible for you to be deficient in protein.[6]

To keep your body running efficiently, greens are one of the most important food groups. Green vegetables are among the most nutrient-dense of all foods and are full of alkaline minerals, including calcium, chlorophyll and amino acids. They make up your key Beauty Foods that regenerate and purify your cells.

Besides greens, you want to eat substantial portions of a wide range of vegetables, which will supply you with key minerals, enzymes and vitamins. Their fiber will help sweep waste from the body, as well as fill you up.

Your best beauty greens and vegetables include the following:

Artichokes (Jerusalem)	Carrots	Green beans	Romaine lettuce
	Cauliflower	Kale	Scallions
Arugula	Celery	Lamb's quarters	Sea vegetables
Asparagus	Chard	Leeks	Shallots
Beans	Chives	Mushrooms	Spinach
Beet greens	Cilantro	Mustard greens	Sprouts (all varieties)
Beets	Collard greens	Okra	
Bok choy	Dandelion greens	Onions	Sweet potatoes
Broccoli	Dill	Parsley	Swiss chard
Brussels sprouts	Endive	Parsnips	Turnips
Cabbage (green, purple or Chinese)	Escarole	Peppers	Watercress
	Frisée	Radishes	Wheatgrass

It's preferable to eat only fresh vegetables. However, frozen vegetables are the next best choice if you don't have access to fresh produce or the time to purchase it. Canned vegetables should be avoided altogether, as they may contain preservatives or chemicals such as bisphenol A, are high in sodium and tend to have lower nutritional value than fresh or frozen vegetables.

Why Organic Matters

A study conducted in 2002 by Rutgers University revealed an astonishing difference in mineral content between organic and conventional produce, especially in terms of the minerals iron, calcium, magnesium, manganese and potassium. The Rutgers research found 87 percent more trace elements and minerals in organic produce versus produce that was commercially grown.[7]

Not only is organic food possibly more nutritious, since it tends to be grown in better-quality soil, it also doesn't contain the noxious pesticides used in conventional farming. Pesticides are neurotoxins that destroy the central nervous system of various pests. Whenever you eat conventionally grown produce, you invariably eat trace pesticides, as well. Exposure to these pesticides may contribute to a whole host of health problems, such as cancer, birth defects, damage to the central nervous system and developmental problems.[8]

If you're on a budget and need to prioritize organic purchases, the Environmental Working Group's list of the "Dirty Dozen" is especially useful. The group analyzes data from the Department of Agriculture to determine which produce contains the most pesticide residue. EWG estimates that you can reduce your pesticide exposure by a whopping 80 percent if you switch to organic when buying these twelve foods:[9]

Apples	Spinach	Potatoes
Celery	Nectarines	Blueberries
Strawberries	Grapes	Lettuce
Peaches	Sweet bell peppers	Kale/collard greens

Clean food equals clean bodies, which equal clean, natural beauty. It's as simple as that. If you can't buy all organic produce, don't let that deter you from eating vegetables and following the program. Look into the various fruit and vegetable cleansers in the produce section of health food stores or you can soak your produce for thirty minutes to an hour in a mixture of filtered water and $3/4$ cup of apple cider vinegar. This can at least help to reduce some of the pesticide content, though, of course, it won't help increase the mineral content of produce.

EAT MORE RAW THAN COOKED VEGETABLES

Eating vegetables raw is the key to obtaining the most beautifying vitamins, enzymes and nutrition, so eat plenty of salads and raw veggies every day. Any type of heat will destroy some of their nutrients. But I know it's not reasonable to eat only salads all the time. It's okay to have some cooked vegetables, especially when you're transitioning and when eating dinner. When cooking vegetables, avoid charring or overboiling them, because you want to preserve the nutrients as much as you can. Steaming or lightly cooking in a bit of vegetable broth, for example, will retain some of the vegetables' nutrients and ensure they are digested easily.

Drink Water *between* Meals, Not *at* Meals

You've heard how important it is to stay hydrated, and that you need pure, filtered water. However, when you start eating the Beauty Detox way, you will be getting water from lots of water-containing fruits and vegetables, so you may not need to adhere to the general recommendation of eight full glasses of water a day. Individualize and drink the amount your body needs, which is also dictated by your activity level and the climate you live in.

It's important to drink water when you wake up and throughout the morning so that you start your day hydrated. Just by ensuring you are hydrated will give you more energy.

Drink significant quantities of water at least half an hour before your meals or an hour following meals. During mealtimes, drink as little as possible. Too much liquid with meals dilutes your digestive juices and can slow digestion considerably. What happens when digestion is delayed? It contributes to the dreaded sludge. Think of a stagnant pond (your food and lots of liquids mixed together in your stomach) versus a waterfall (the liquid on its own), which efficiently and continuously flows. The pond scenario isn't going to promote your beauty.

Also get in the habit of squeezing some liver-supporting, vitamin C–filled lemon in your water for an added benefit.

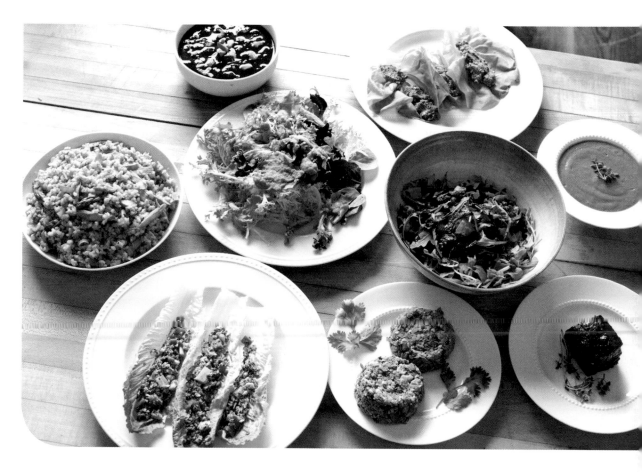

LIMIT ANIMAL PROTEIN

Over the past decade or so, a number of high-protein, low-carb diets have become increasingly popular. A study published in 2002[10] and funded by the Atkins Center for Complementary Medicine researched fifty-one obese people who were put on the low-carb Atkins Diet.[11] Over six months, forty-one subjects maintained the diet and lost an average of twenty pounds. Sounds good, doesn't it? But consider that the participants in the study were consuming an average of only 1,450 calories per day, which is 35 percent less than the average American consumption of 2,250 calories a day. On any kind of diet, if you were to restrict your calories by at least 35 percent, you would lose weight, at least for the short term. In the same study the researchers also stated that "at some point during the twenty-four weeks, 68% reported constipation, 63% reported bad breath, 51% reported headaches, 10% reported hair loss, and one woman reported increased menstrual bleeding."[12]

Another frightening figure from the study is that dieters had a fifty-three percent increase in the amount of calcium excreted in their urine, which is a big problem for bone density and health. A diet that creates such high levels of constipation shows how unnatural it is for the human body. Constipation holds toxins in the body and is incredibly aging.

Digesting animal protein creates all sorts of by-products in the body, like purines, uric acid and ammonia by-products. These toxins are absorbed into your bloodstream through the colon and circulate all around your body. When your blood is clogged with toxins, it can't transport as many beautifying minerals, and these toxins can age and clog the skin cells of your face. Furthermore, excessive protein consumption overworks the liver and kidneys.[13] In his book *Conscious Eating,* Gabriel Cousens, M.D., discusses how ammonia, a by-product of digesting protein, contributes to aging. As he notes, "Ammonia, which is a breakdown product of a high-flesh-food diet, is directly toxic to the system. It has been found to create free radical damage and cross-linking (a process associated with skin wrinkles and aging), as well as depletes the body's energy."[14]

Ketosis, which may occur as a result of a low-carb diet, whereby by-products called ketones accumulate in your body, makes the blood acidic.[15] An acidic body tends to age faster. Take a look for yourself at people who are on high-protein, low-carb diets. They usually look "hardened" and far older than they are, with what I call the "old skinny" look, which has lost all its youthfulness. I'll bet you can think of some "old skinny" people!

One study published in the *Asia Pacific Journal of Clinical Nutrition* focusing on the short- and long-term effects of high-protein and low-carb diets found that "complications such as heart arrhythmias, cardiac contractile function impairment, sudden death, osteo-porosis, kidney damage, increased cancer risk, impairment of physical activity and lipid abnormalities can all be linked to long-term restriction of carbohydrates in the diet."[16] Animal protein is also the most complex of all foods: it takes about twice as long as other foods to pass through your digestive system.[17] The more slowly a food is digested in your body, which is a hot 98.6 degrees, the greater the chance that toxins can be created.

There definitely have to be limits to the amount of concentrated protein you consume. The "eat as much animal protein as you can" theory is both aging to your skin and body, and dangerous. Taking in more protein than is needed places a heavy burden on your body, creating acidity (see Chapter 2 for more info on acidity) and wasting Beauty Energy—the very thing you are trying to avoid.

Many people love eating meat, so you may choose not to become a full vegetarian. You don't have to give it up completely if you don't want to, so long as you stick to these tips when you consume animal protein:

◉ **Buy organic, hormone-free meat, preferably from a local farm or source.** The ugly truth is that factory-farmed animals are fed copious amounts of chemicals, hormones, antibiotics and steroids before being slaughtered, and all these toxins wind up on your plate and in your body. A report in 2001 by the Union of Concerned Scientists, coauthored by Margaret Mellon, Ph.D., J.D., director of the organization's Food and Environment Program, examined the use of antibiotics in farmed animals. In a press statement, Dr. Mellon said, "Our report finds that there are twenty-five million pounds of antibiotics used in cattle, swine and poultry for nontherapeutic purposes, including growth promotion and disease prevention. The breakdown is about four million pounds in cattle, almost eleven million pounds in swine and ten million pounds in poultry. By contrast, the report finds only three million pounds of antibiotics are used in human medicine. That means we're using eight times the amount of antibiotics in healthy animals as we're using to treat diseases in our children and ourselves."[18] These alarmingly high levels of antibiotics in the food supply can contribute to antibiotic resistance in humans, not to mention many other health concerns associated with continually consuming antibiotics.

◉ **Eat animal protein once a day at most, and eat it at dinnertime.** Eating any type of animal protein more than once a day will make your body too acidic, and will require far too much energy to efficiently digest the more complex protein chains. And avoid eating animal protein until dinner (which ideally should be at least a few hours before bedtime) so that your Beauty Energy is not wasted during the day and can be freed up for cleansing, weight loss and creating beauty. Eventually, your goal should be to limit the consumption of meat to two to three times per week at most.

The Lowdown on Fish

Fish and seafood are generally good nutritional choices. But that's not to say that you should start loading up on seafood. Fish is cited as one of the most polluted foods you can eat. Three of the biggest water contaminants that are found in fish are hydrocarbons, PCBs and mercury, although there are others like DDT and fertilizers in our waters.

The sad fact is that our water sources, including the oceans, lakes and rivers, have been polluted with megadoses of toxic chemicals, and fish today act as a sponge for toxins and are often heavily contaminated. Toxins diminish your beauty and age you faster, so although some will argue that fish has some positive health benefits, such as good omega-3 oils (which we'll discuss later; there are cleaner options for getting these fats), the benefits have to be balanced against the dangers.

The American College of Obstetricians and Gynecologists[19] and the American Academy of Pediatrics[20] recommend strict limits on fish consumption for pregnant women because of risks posed to the developing fetus. However, especially if you eat out at restaurants for dinner and can choose from some better options (see below), you may choose to keep fish in your diet as part of your moderate amount of weekly animal protein intake.

Here are some tips for choosing fish if you would like to eat it:

- Don't eat fish or seafood more than a maximum of two times a week.

- Choose fish that may be lower in heavy metals and toxins: wild Alaskan salmon, mahi-mahi, sole, tilapia, trout, striped sea bass, haddock, halibut and whitefish.[21]

- Avoid fish high in toxins: swordfish, tuna, shark, bluefish, Chilean sea bass, tilefish, marlin, shellfish (which is particularly high in the heavy metal cadmium) such as shrimp and blue crab, Atlantic or farmed salmon, bluefish, wild striped bass, mackerel and grouper.[22]

- Avoid store-bought canned tuna fish, which is high in mercury. A woman who eats just one can of tuna a week will be 30 percent over the EPA cut-off for safe mercury levels.[23]

- Because a lot of the chemicals are stored in the fish's fat, be sure to broil or bake your fish to allow as much fat as possible to drain from it. When eating out, order baked fish as opposed to pan-seared or fried dishes.

- Be cautious when eating sushi and sashimi. If the fish weren't toxic, it would be a great choice since it's raw, and the amino acids that make up the fish proteins don't become denatured from cooking. But tuna, salmon and other fish commonly used for sushi and sashimi are often the most toxic fish of all.

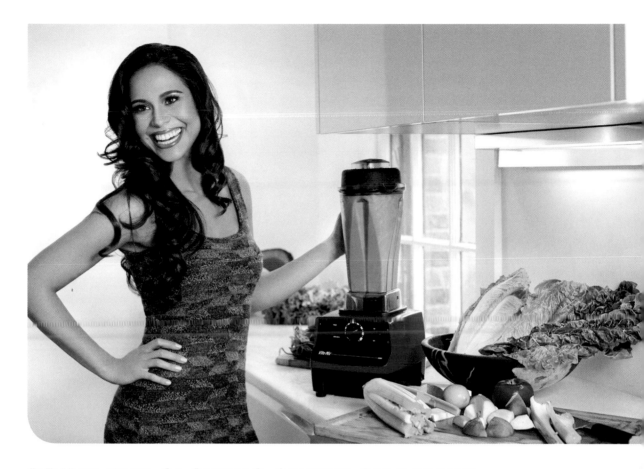

DRINK THE GLOWING GREEN SMOOTHIE (OR JUICE) EVERY DAY

My superfoods aren't exotic, expensive, or hard-to-find fruits or plants from foreign countries. Instead, green-based drinks, the Glowing Green Smoothie and Glowing Green Juice (see pages 168 and 172), are the real super foods. These green drinks are delicious, because lemon, fruit and/or stevia cut right through any "green" taste and make for a balanced, enjoyable flavor. You will be pleasantly surprised with your first sip. When I drink them, I get a rush of sustained energy that lasts for hours, I feel clearheaded and calm, and it's much easier to focus on work or any tasks at hand. My skin has started to glow since making the drinks a regular part of my life (hence the name of the drinks). I can't wait for you to experience the same thing! The great news is that as the biochemistry of your body changes and your skin, body and energy start to improve, you will actually look forward to your Glowing Green drinks. I have had so many clients report back weeks or months after they start that they are now addicted to their green-drink ritual.

Think having a blended vegetable drink sounds weird? Don't want to invest in a blender at this time? It's totally okay. In the Blossoming Beauty Phase in Chapter 3, you will not absolutely have to make or consume these green drinks. The Blossoming Beauty Phase still provides for powerful cleansing and improvement by incorporating all the principles in Chapters 1 and 2. Down the road, as you start to experience great results and your body becomes cleaner, you may be interested in going further and revisiting the Glowing Green drinks, which come into play in the Radiant Beauty Phase.

Perhaps you are thinking, *How many days a week do I have to do that?* or *For how long do I have to that?* And my question back to you is, "How many days do you want to be healthy and beautiful?" This is not a quick-fix answer to detoxification but a way to permanently break out of your old habits and improve your health and beauty for the long term. To maximize your intake of minerals and enzymes, aim to consume the Glowing Green Smoothie or Glowing Green Juice every day, or at least five times a week.

THE GLOWING GREEN SMOOTHIE

I've been talking about my Glowing Green Smoothie on my website, www.kimberlysnyder.net, and in the press for years. Many of my clients and readers fondly refer to it as the "GGS." By blending foods before eating them, you "predigest" them, so the body does not have to work to break down the foods and waste unnecessary energy in digestion.

Many of the important minerals and other nutrients in food are encased in the cell walls, and these need to be ruptured to extract the nutrients. Thus, blending helps make the greens' full spectrum of nutrition readily available to the body without the body doing any work. You also add some fresh fruit, which really balances the taste of the greens and adds powerful antioxidants and vitamins. Served cold, the Glowing Green Smoothie (see the recipe on page 168) is delicious.

What is so wonderful about the Glowing Green Smoothie is that you retain the integrity of the whole vegetables and fruits, so you still enjoy all the fiber. In nature, fruits and veggies contain both juice *and* fiber, and I firmly believe that you cannot improve on nature. I believe in eating whole foods, and the Glowing Green Smoothie is made of whole foods in their full nutritional package, simply broken down by blending. When you move into this new way of eating, fiber is one of your best friends, as it helps to sweep out the newly awakened poisons and helps strengthen your bowel movements. Increased fiber is one of the most important ways to continuously cleanse your body.

Besides many other functions, the liver can pump excessive fat out of the body through the bile into the small intestines. If the diet is high in fiber, which you can boost daily with the Glowing Green Smoothie, this unwanted fat will be carried out of the body, which will reduce the recirculation of fat and toxins and help with weight loss (good!). If the diet is low in fiber, some of the fat and toxins can recirculate back to the liver, via enterohepatic circulation (the circulation of fluids between gut and liver), and will not leave the body (not good!).

The high volume of fiber in the Glowing Green Smoothie also keeps you feeling fuller throughout the morning and up to lunch, especially in the beginning, when you are used to being stimulated by denser and heavier volumes of food. The other advantage of the Glowing Green Smoothie over Glowing Green Juice is that the whole foods are blended rather than pulverized and extracted into a juice, which keeps them from oxidizing as quickly. For this reason, the smoothie can be stored in your fridge for a few days, whereas you should ideally drink a fresh-pressed juice within fifteen minutes after juicing. (Special cold-pressed juicers can retain the enzymes of a juice for longer periods.)

Nix the Caffeine

Caffeine is absorbed throughout the body and affects many of your critical organs, interfering with numerous processes in the body. Caffeine is particularly taxing on the liver, which has to metabolize it. Too much caffeine can overload the liver and slow down the liver's ability to burn fat efficiently and cleanse other toxins from your system. Caffeine can also contribute to increased levels of cortisol, a stress hormone that has been linked to excess fat storage, especially around the belly. Caffeine can promote norepinephrine production, which is another stress hormone that affects your brain and nervous system, raising your heart rate and blood pressure. It creates that jittery feeling you may be familiar with after having even just one or two cups of coffee.

This is one of the reasons I don't recommend drinking much green tea, and why I personally avoid it. Even though green tea contains some healthy antioxidants, one cup has around thirty-five milligrams of caffeine. White tea, with only about eight milligrams of caffeine per cup—or better yet, caffeine-free rooibos tea and herbal teas—are much better choices, and they contain antioxidants, such as aspalathin and nothofagin.

GLOWING GREEN JUICE

I consider the modern-day father of Glowing Green Juice to be Dr. Norman Walker, who lived to be well over one hundred. Glowing Green Juice is loaded with enzymes, oxygen, minerals and vitamins that, according to Dr. Walker, have been "liberated" from the other food components and can be easily absorbed into the intestinal wall.

Glowing Green Juice comes into play in the True Beauty Phase (see Chapter 3), after you've made other necessary adjustments. In True Beauty, you will consume both the Glowing Green Smoothie and Glowing Green Juice, depending on that day's meal plan. Glowing Green Juice is pure liquid nutrition that will fuel your body. As you cleanse and become more alkaline, you need less stimulation from solid food in general.

Glowing Green Juice is not made from whole foods anymore in their natural state; the foods are processed by the juicing process and stripped of their fiber. Since it lacks fiber, Glowing Green Juice may not be as satisfying or keep you full for longer periods the way the Glowing Green Smoothie does. Many people, even at the True Beauty stage, skip the Glowing Green Juice and stick with the Glowing Green Smoothie permanently, as they personally prefer it and feel more of an energy boost from it. Personally, I regularly consume both, but I do not skip my fiber-filled Glowing Green Smoothie, which is my first love, and Glowing Green Juice is a snack sometimes later in the day.

You might be wondering about the juices or smoothies available in stores. V8 Naked and all the other prepackaged, prebottled commercial drinks simply don't count. The nature of the bottling process means that the juices have been pasteurized, and that means the vegetables and fruits have been heated to such high temperatures that the enzymes and much of the nutrition have been killed and denatured. Juices should be pressed and consumed fresh to realize their enzyme and nutritional benefits. However, there are some special cold-pressed juicers that can retain the enzymes and nutrients of fruits and vegetables for a day or two, so long as these juices are stored cold and aren't pasteurized.

VARYING YOUR GLOWING GREEN DRINKS

The Glowing Green Smoothie can keep in your fridge for up to two to three days, but if it's easier for you from a time standpoint to make larger batches of green drinks and freeze them in portions, that's perfectly fine. Many of my clients do this. Although fresh is ideal, enzymes and other nutrients hold up pretty well in the freezer. Don't worry about losing out on too much by freezing larger batches; you will still get plenty of minerals and nutrients from the drinks. It's more important that you stick to the plan and consume your green drinks every morning, rather than worrying that you could not make the Glowing Green Smoothie from scratch some days.

Remember that the recipes for the Glowing Green Smoothie and Glowing Green Juice are mere guidelines. Many people email me or leave a comment on the Beauty Detox community website, writing something along the lines of, "Ugh! I don't even like to eat cilantro, and now you want me to drink it?" or "Celery makes me want to gag; I can't deal with it." Well, you don't have to. Skip the produce you don't like, simply swapping the celery for something you like (say, cucumber), or just add more of the other greens that are already in there.

Think of your favorite fruits as the opening act of a concert, and your leafy greens as the headliner. The opening band (or fruit, in this case) is really the support for the awesome main act (or leafy greens), which is the most important reason you've come to the show.

Variety will ensure that you get a wide range of the key minerals, since different minerals are present in higher quantities in different greens. As you continue on this plan, you'll be surprised to see that your personal tastes and preferences for different greens will expand as you start to alter the biochemical makeup of your body. I used to think kale was nasty, and avoided arugula at all costs, but now they are two of my staple faves. Who would have thought that would happen? So, remember, as your body changes physically, so do your tastes. Also, choose local, seasonal and organic greens and fruits whenever possible. They don't have to travel very far to reach you, thus reducing the carbon footprint. They will also be richer in minerals, as they have more time to ripen in the field or orchard.

Have a Light Morning

We've all been told that breakfast is the most important meal of the day. According to this old belief, we need to stock up at this important first meal in order to supply ourselves with energy to get going. You may eat breakfast first thing upon waking in the morning or soon after. You may even eat early "for energy" when you are not yet hungry. Your new rule about breakfast is this: never eat when you aren't hungry. If your body is not telling you that you're hungry, it's telling you that it doesn't need any food. We all need to start listening to our bodies more instead of trying to follow any diet "formula."

What you do in the morning is critical for achieving your goals. When you wake up, you have a fresh start. You have not put any new food in your body since the evening before, so your body will go to work eliminating and cleaning out what is already in the system. Through the night (assuming you haven't eaten dinner too late) and the morning may be the only time that your body's energy is not consumed in digesting and can instead be directed to actually cleansing. In the morning, you probably wake up with some pungent body odors—bad breath, a coated tongue—and sleep in your eyes. We can all be too stinky to go out in public without doing something about it first. But all these odors and substances coming up to the surface are the result of various forms of cleansing that your body has employed throughout the night in order to eliminate toxins.

From waking until noon is key for cleansing and achieving complete elimination. The moment you start eating, you shut off the body's cleansing mechanism, and your energy has to be directed to digestion. So give yourself the morning to have a literal clean start, letting the body root out toxins and eliminate waste. When I say *eliminate,* yes, I do mean poop. Don't be embarrassed by us talking about this—pooping is super important! Above all, you don't want to prevent your body from eliminating as much as possible. If you obstruct your body's elimination functions, your body will not be able to thoroughly rid itself of waste matter, which is constantly accumulating. Toxicity will build, weight will pile on and be harder to take off, and your beauty will fade drastically.

Over time, you'll feel so great from eating light earlier in the day that your cravings will greatly subside. I used to be a breakfast girl and would wake up starving in the morning and have big morning feasts. I was able to overcome that habit over time. By sticking to light mornings, I feel infinitely better and more energized throughout my entire day. It's not an exaggeration to say that light mornings have improved my entire life. I see the difference it has made in my body and beauty, from my skin to my hair and nails, not to mention how easy it is to maintain my ideal weight.

Try it out for yourself. See how you feel shifting to lighter breakfasts for three weeks, and then go back to the heavier way of eating breakfast. I'm pretty sure you won't want to go back, though, because you will feel so much better. You'll realize the heavy breakfasts really were making you tired. There is no stronger proof than personal experience.

Of course, some of us like to enjoy the occasional hearty brunch on vacation or on the weekend with friends or family. Don't worry. You won't have to ban brunch forever; your body can deal with the occasional off-wagon event. What you want to focus on are everyday habits and patterns that you repeat over and over again.

GIVE UP DAIRY

I usually stress moderation with all food groups, including fish and other animal protein, if you really want to keep them in your diet. However, there is the one category where there is no room for moderation: cut out the dairy. Period. Work to either eliminate dairy from your diet immediately or transition it out completely over time. As Elson M. Haas, M.D., states in his nutritional tome *Staying Healthy with Nutrition,* "Lifelong use of milk is among the biggest misconceptions and mistakes in nutrition."[24]

You won't find any other species on the planet, except for humans, drinking milk past the infancy stage, and none (except humans) consume the milk of another animal. Pause, and really think about that. This practice could not be more contrary to the inherent laws of nature.

You may be thinking, *Hey, how come I've always heard I should drink milk for calcium? And aren't skim milk and yogurt healthy?* You have heard these things because dairy is a big business. With hundreds of millions of people consuming dairy every day, there is a lot of money to be made by this industry, which in turn also puts a lot of money into guaranteeing that certain health claims are widely disseminated, down to providing educational material about the "benefits" of dairy products for children.

THE PROBLEM IS CASEIN

The main protein in cow's milk is casein, making up 87 percent of cow's milk protein.[25] The other protein in milk is whey, which makes up a much smaller amount.

There are so many thousands of studies on the detrimental effects of dairy, but the strongest argument I can share with you is that of all animal proteins, casein is the one that most consistently and strongly seems to promote cancer. The long-term, in-depth research of the China Study, which was funded by such prestigious organizations as the National Institutes of Health, the American Cancer Society and the American Institute for Cancer Research, found a strong correlation between casein intake and the promotion of cancer cell growth when exposed to carcinogens. Dr. T. Colin Campbell, a professor in the Division of Nutritional Sciences at Cornell University, studied the effect of diet and carcinogen exposure and found a strong correlation between protein intake and cancer growth. Of all the proteins he studied, Dr. Campbell found that casein most "consistently and strongly promoted cancer" and that it "promoted all stages of the cancer process."[26]

There is some casein present in human breast milk, but in cow's milk there is 300 percent more,[27] helping cows develop huge bones. Casein is such a strong binder that it has been used as an ingredient in wood glue. Without the necessary enzymes, such as lactase, to break it down, casein coagulates in the stomach and is very difficult for your body to break down. When casein does break down in the human stomach, it produces casomorphins, which are peptides, or protein fragments, that have an *opioid effect,* meaning they act like opiates in the brain, causing a slightly euphoric effect—a troublesome effect considering how unhealthy casein really is. Some studies hypothesize that casomorphin (from casein) can cause or aggravate autism.[28] Dairy has also been found to double the risk of prostate cancer: a Harvard review of research from 2001 found that "men with the highest dairy intakes had approximately double the risk of total prostate cancer, and up to a fourfold increase in risk of metastatic or fatal prostate cancer relative to low consumers."[29]

The Yogurt Myth

I'm constantly asked about yogurt, which is widely advertised as a health food. But let's look at the facts: it contains casein, it's pasteurized and it's mucus-forming. World-renowned surgeon Dr. Hiromi Shinya, chief of the Surgical Endoscopy Unit at Beth Israel Medical Center and clinical professor of surgery at Albert Einstein College of Medicine, has examined the stomachs and intestines of hundreds of thousands of patients, and has performed over 370,000 colonoscopies.[30] Calling it a common myth that eating yogurt every day improves digestion, Dr. Shinya states in *The Enzyme Factor* that, "I have yet to meet a person who eats yogurt on a daily basis and still has good intestinal health."[31]

Yogurt is marketed as being good for preventing constipation and helping people lose weight, mainly due to the lactobacilli it contains. Dr. Shinya hypothesizes that the reason people feel that yogurt is curing constipation is because the yogurt isn't digested properly. It therefore results in indigestion, and that causes people to develop milk diarrhea to excrete it out of the colon. This excretion of some matter is what people mistakenly believe is improving their colon's health. As he states, "Your intestine's condition will worsen if you eat yogurt every day."

Note: I am a huge proponent of probiotic-rich foods from nondairy sources. Check out more info on this in Chapter 2, and see my list of yogurt replacements on page 27.

THEN THERE'S MUCUS

Dairy has another downside: mucus. Despite its rather revolting name, mucus is actually a natural secretion that your body produces to protect the surfaces of membranes. It's clear and slippery, and it coats anything you ingest. Where mucus starts to be problematic is when you have too much of it. Mucus engulfs toxins and the toxic remnants of certain foods, and can become thick and cloudy to "trap" the toxicity and help it leave the body.[32]

Excessive mucus can begin to harden and build up along the walls of your intestines, adding to the sludge and slowing down matter moving through the intestinal tract. And dairy is one of the most mucus-forming foods there is.

When you ingest milk, cheese and other dairy products, it puts a huge burden on the body to try to get rid of the mucus. Dairy products begin to wreak havoc on your body as soon as they are ingested, so your body then tries desperately to get rid of them in different ways, such as through phlegm, mucus or pimples. Because dairy products are so acid-forming, clogging and difficult to digest, consistently eating them will not help you lose the extra weight in those troublesome areas—your belly, upper arms, thighs, hips and under your chin. Dairy ultimately keeps you from reaching your true beauty potential. As you start to cut dairy out of your system, your body will start to clear out the mucus caused by the dairy. Pounds will fall off, your skin will start to clear and your beauty will start to radiate.

BUT WHAT ABOUT CALCIUM?

You've heard that you need to consume calcium in order to build strong bones and prevent diseases like osteoporosis. The best way, you've always been told, to get your calcium is from dairy products. But statistics show that bone issues like osteoporosis and hip fractures are *more* frequent in populations where dairy is highly consumed and calcium consumption is generally high.[33] American women drink thirty to thirty-two times as much cow's milk as New Guineans, but suffer forty-seven times as many broken hips. An analysis conducted on multiple countries showed a high statistical association between dairy consumption and higher rates of hip fractures.[34] One study out of the Yale School of Medicine in 1992 analyzed the link between protein intake and fracture rates in women fifty years of age and older from sixteen different countries. The study found that the consumption of animal protein was associated with 70 percent of the fractures in the women studied.[35]

From his extensive research for the China Study, Dr. T. Colin Campbell reported in the *New York Times* that there was basically no osteoporosis in China, yet the average calcium intake there was 544 mg per day, as compared with 1,143 mg per day in the United States, which was mostly derived from dairy sources.[36]

Numerous studies show the same correlation: the more protein consumed, the more calcium lost. So what's going on? Cow's milk does, in fact, have a lot of calcium in it, but much of it is not easily assimilated or used by the body. There is a lot of phosphorus in dairy products, and it binds to the calcium in your digestive tract and makes most of the calcium impossible to absorb. In addition, dairy products are extremely acidic to the body, and the increased acid load in the body causes you to lose calcium from your bones, since calcium is an alkaline mineral and neutralizes the acidity. (See more on the topic of alkalinity in Chapter 2.)

Don't be fooled into looking at a label and being impressed by how much calcium a dairy product contains. You'll end up with a net loss of calcium after digestion. Focus on eating more alkaline-forming plant foods, which will provide calcium and won't cause it to be leached from your body. The best sources for calcium are dark, leafy, green vegetables, as well as sea vegetables, nuts and seeds (see the Oxalic Acid discussion on page 94). Here's a list of your best plant sources of calcium:

Almonds	Dates	Sesame seeds (and tahini, which is made from sesame seeds)
Bok choy	Figs	
Broccoli	Kale	Spinach
Cactus (Nopales)	Oranges	Sunflower seeds
Cauliflower	Romaine lettuce	Turnip greens
Collard greens	Sea vegetables	Watercress
Cucumber		

FINDING DAIRY ALTERNATIVES

I stress the importance of transitioning throughout this book, and part of that is finding alternatives to your favorite foods to make it easier and tastier to eat yourself beautiful.

Cheese lovers, I have great news for you: goat's milk and goat's cheese are far better options than cow's milk and cow's milk products. The natural enzymes in a goat are closer to those in humans than those in cows, and you can digest goat's milk exponentially better. If you love cheese, you'll be thrilled to know that you can switch to goat's milk cheese as an occasional treat. It's best to consume goat's milk cheese in its raw, unpasteurized form, although even pasteurized goat's milk cheese is still better than pasteurized cow's milk products. Sheep's milk cheese is the next best choice as it may be easier to digest than cow's milk products, but it is high in fat.

Here are some other, healthier foods that mimic your favorite dairy products:

MILK

Almond milk	Hemp milk
Coconut milk	Rice milk (a low-nutrient choice that is my last recommendation in this category)

CHEESE

Seed cheese or other nonsoy vegan alternatives	Pasteurized goat's milk cheese or pasteurized sheep's milk cheese (not ideal choices, as the pasteurization makes these products clogging)
Raw goat's milk cheese or raw sheep's milk cheese (these do contain lactose)	Raw cow's milk cheese (the least favorable choice)

YOGURT

Probiotic & Enzyme Salad (see Part III)	A daily probiotic (see Chapter 2)
Kimchi (see Part III)	Goat's milk kefir (I consider the other options cleaner and superior to this choice; this will be pasteurized unless made or purchased fresh from a farm)
Coconut yogurt, store-bought or homemade (see Part III)	

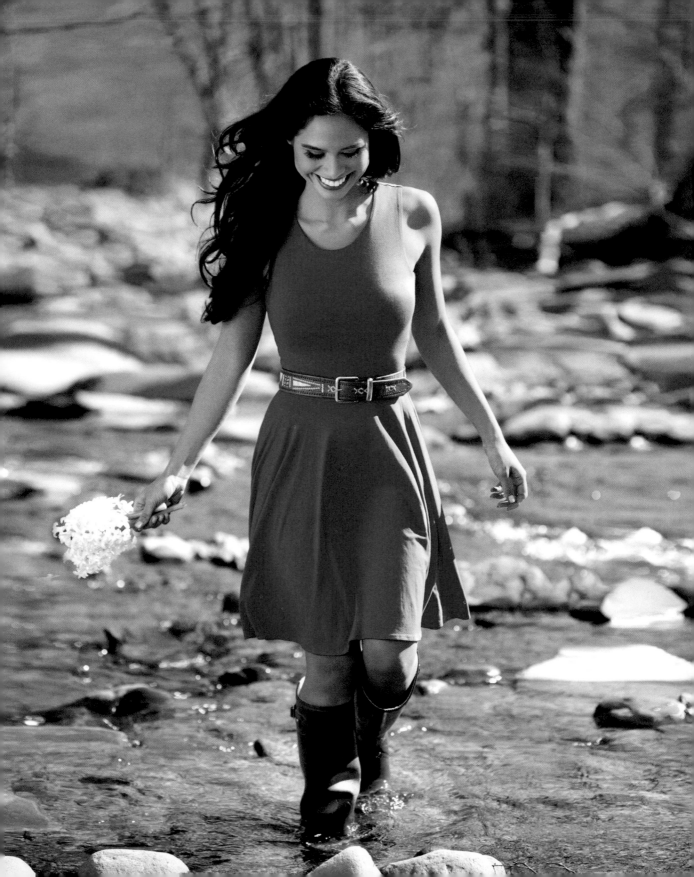

ADDITIONAL BEAUTY DETOX PRINCIPLES

2

Now that you understand the basic Beauty Detox concepts—eat more veggies and fewer animal products, drink the Glowing Green Smoothie or Juice every day and give up dairy—you can begin to think about other guidelines to add over time. These include:

- Incorporating ongoing cleansing
- Eating fruit on an empty stomach
- Eating high-alkaline foods
- Eating beautiful carbohydrates and starches
- Eating more plant protein
- Avoiding most soy products
- Eating beauty fats in moderation
- Getting your beauty minerals and enzymes

Each is covered in its own section in this chapter.

INCORPORATE ONGOING CLEANSING

As you start to incorporate the primary Beauty Detox principles, this one is the next most important one to incorporate. Why? Because ongoing cleansing is one of the most important ways to ensure that beauty nutrients are made available to your cells, so you can achieve your full beauty potential, reverse aging and lose weight. In fact, it might just be *the* most important way. If you have changed your diet but are still not getting the results you are after, it is most likely because you are not cleansing enough. When you hear the word "cleanse," you may think in terms of a noun—doing "a cleanse," which is usually some kind of fasting or herbal program for a few days here and there, a few times a year. While certain, properly conducted programs can be useful in getting you back on track, the most important thing is to change that mind-set and think of cleansing as a verb, and accelerate and initiate cleans*ing* on an ongoing basis.

PROBIOTIC & ENZYME SALAD

Although fermented foods are a critical food group in many cultures, such as Korea with its kimchi, Germany with its sauerkraut and France with its *choucroute*, the traditional American diet and the modern Western diet in general are sorely lacking in raw versions of these foods, which is a real shame. My Probiotic & Enzyme Salad (see page 212) is designed to make up for this lack. It is made of raw, fermented vegetables, mainly cabbage, that have been chopped and left in airtight glass containers at room temperature for several days. This allows the beneficial *lactobacilli* and enzymes that are already naturally present in the vegetables to flourish, creating a food that is extremely rich in probiotics (friendly bacteria), enzymes and minerals. It's really raw sauerkraut, but when you hear that word, you may think of the soggy, salty food that is sold at hot dog stands or in supermarkets as a condiment for hot dogs or Wiener schnitzel. That is not what I'm talking about here. Commercial sauerkraut is loaded with refined salt and pasteurized to high temperatures, which destroys its important benefits. Raw sauerkraut, on the other hand, is a powerful source of probiotics and enzymes—two essentials for healthy digestion, improved Beauty Energy and ongoing cleansing.

Years ago a friend from a yoga studio in New York City told me about a farm with a table at the Union Square farmers' market that sells delicious raw sauerkraut and other cultured vegetables. Since I frequent that farmers' market several times a week, I decided to check it out. I had studied the benefits of cultured foods and had tried some of Dr. Ann Wigmore's rejuvelac recipe, a drink made from fermenting quinoa or cabbage, but I had really never consumed cultured foods on a regular basis to truly experience the incredible benefits.

I loved the taste immediately, and I began to pile raw sauerkraut on my daily dinner salads and sometimes also had it at lunch. I also found that if I happened to be eating grains, like millet, or a protein dish, like a nut pâté, the raw sauerkraut greatly helped me digest the other foods. I had more energy and, yes, I was eliminating much more frequently. Exciting stuff!

I am now convinced that raw, cultured vegetables are among the most important foods of our modern day. As they are powerful, extremely helpful weapons to clean out sludge and to look younger and more radiant, I like calling these raw, fermented veggies Probiotic & Enzyme Salad, so that you are reminded of their key benefits.

As the inner balance of good bacteria is restored in your body, you'll be better able to shed excess weight. Your skin will improve. Your energy will become more vibrant. Because these functions are so important, you must consume Probiotic & Enzyme Salad regularly in addition to taking a probiotic supplement and digestive enzymes. You may wonder, *Why can't I just pop a pill and be done with it?* Because Probiotic & Enzyme Salad is a whole food, and our best strategy with probiotics and enzymes is to combine whole foods with supplements. Probiotic & Enzyme Salad also helps you digest other foods you eat and may help balance various cravings.

Although you can buy raw, cultured veggies in health food stores (look for jars of raw sauerkraut in the refrigerated section), they are very easy and inexpensive to prepare in large batches at home, to ensure you can enjoy them regularly. You can also control how much sodium you ingest, as store-bought brands tend to have excessive amounts of salt. All it takes is a little bit of time to chop and store. And it's completely worth the benefits that come with regularly consuming these veggies. Consuming one-half to one cup with dinner at least five nights a week would be ideal. Make them part of your life, as I have. Check out the recipe for Probiotic & Enzyme Salad in Part III. With some planning, you should have these foods available to you in your own refrigerator for the cost of a few cents a day.

PSST... A BIG BEAUTY SECRET: PROBIOTICS

Probiotics may help restore your internal balance and increase your vibrancy and overall health in the following ways:

- ◉ Improve digestive functions, helping to eliminate constipation and diarrhea
- ◉ Improve liver function
- ◉ Improve resistance to allergies
- ◉ Improve vitamin synthesis, and specifically the manufacturing of B vitamins
- ◉ Increase energy
- ◉ Improve the absorption of nutrients
- ◉ Help eliminate bloating and heartburn

I wholeheartedly recommend taking a good probiotic every day. Probiotics help preserve a healthy digestive environment and play a critical role in your immune system, 80 percent of which resides in your gut. Adults have around 400 different species and strains of friendly bacteria in their digestive tracts. When you're healthy, you have 80 to 85 percent friendly bacteria. When there is an overbalance of unfriendly bacteria in your system and the percentage of friendly bacteria diminishes, it creates a condition known as dysbiosis.

When it comes to choosing a probiotic supplement, keep in mind there are numerous probiotics available in the marketplace, and they're all labeled as "probiotics." However, many of them aren't as effective as they could or should be. The benefits of probiotics are realized only when the live probiotic cells make their way to the intestine. The harsh environment of the human stomach kills a good portion of the live cells before they can reach the intestine and benefit your health. So when shopping for a probiotic, look for one that has a specialized delivery system designed to support the safe transport of live cells into the intestine. Also, it's important that there is not just a high culture count overall, but that there's a high culture count of a variety of highly beneficial strains. *Lactobacillus acidophilus* is a common strain and is particularly useful in getting candidiasis under control. *Bifidobacterium bifidum* promotes general immunity. Check out the online resources section at www.kimberlysnyder.net for brands I recommend, as well as where to buy them.

Yogurt and Kefir

As I've already discussed in "The Yogurt Myth," page 24, I don't recommend consuming yogurt. It is made of pasteurized dairy milk, making it a clogging food, and has high levels of the protein casein (see Chapter 1). Even so, many people look to yogurt and kefir as sources of probiotics. But there really is no point in eating yogurt if you're taking a daily probiotic and regularly eating Probiotic & Enzyme Salad and other recipes with cultured ingredients found in Part III. If you can find raw goat's milk kefir (which may be difficult to obtain), that would be an acceptable choice and easier to digest than any cow's milk products, although the other yogurt alternatives I mention on page 27 are better options.

ANOTHER BEAUTY SECRET: DIGESTIVE ENZYMES

Over the years, your enzyme reserve becomes diminished, which means that your body may not be digesting foods as well as it did when you were a child. Any amount of poorly digested food ferments and putrefies in the digestive tract, stimulating the growth of unfriendly bacteria and the creation of toxic, acidic by-products and waste, which then become absorbed into the blood and deposited in tissues all around the body, especially soft-tissue areas, such as the joints.[1] Toxins in the blood also negatively affect your skin and physical appearance. Supplemental digestive enzymes are a critical aid, though they certainly do not replace eating raw plant foods. They can be taken daily and should be ingested right before any meal that contains cooked food. Here are some of the potential benefits of digestive enzymes:

- Improve the absorption and assimilation of minerals and nutrients
- Help to slow the aging process by preserving the body's own enzymes
- Promote efficient digestion
- Free up Beauty Energy to rebuild and replace damaged cells, including the collagen of the skin
- Increase energy
- Enhance cleansing, which can improve acne and other imbalances
- Decrease bloating, gassiness and constipation

If you've never purchased a digestive enzyme supplement, look for "digestive enzyme" on the label—it's near the vitamins at a health food or whole food store. Plant enzymes may be more active at a fuller pH range than animal-based enzymes, so look for one that's vegan and plant-based, rather than one that contains enzymes from bovine animals (cows or oxen) or other animals or animal products. Choose a supplement that contains a blend of lipase, amylase and protease to help efficiently digest fats, starches and proteins. Cellulase is another category of digestive enzymes and can also be useful in a supplement, as it breaks down cellulose and chitin, a fiber similar to cellulose that is found in the cell wall of candida.[2] Check out the online resources section of www.kimberlysnyder.net for recommended brands.

GRAVITY-CENTERED COLONICS

Your colon is the sewer system of the body. When your colon becomes overloaded, toxicity builds in other parts of your body, including your liver and kidneys. When you clean the colon, you start a chain reaction of cleansing the other organs throughout the whole body.

Colonics are a professional procedure that cost about $50 to $125. Although they are somewhat pricey, I firmly believe that properly administered colonics (emphasis on *properly)* are one of the greatest cleansing methods available. With a gravity-centered colonic, water is administered into the rectum by a speculum with split tubing, which simultaneously allows clean water to flow into the colon while waste flows out of the body and directly into the sewage.

Okay, I know it doesn't sound like fun. But having a colonic is like having the underside of your car power-washed for forty-five minutes, and it shouldn't hurt or feel excessively uncomfortable. The gentle pressure of warm water helps dissolve old waste from the walls of your colon and takes it right out. This old sludge in your digestive tract must be removed to allow you to reach your full beauty potential. Even if you go to the bathroom a lot, you will be shocked at how much waste your body can and does hold in your colon, which has the ability to expand and store increasing amounts of garbage. Remember: your body is a hot 98.6 degrees, and all that impacted toxic waste can really bake in there.

Some people think colonics are "bad" because they can wash out some friendly bacteria from your digestive tract. But rest assured that any friendly bacteria that might be removed are easily replaced with a daily probiotic supplement and the consumption of Probiotic & Enzyme Salad.

Gravity-centered colonics typically don't cause major discomfort from having to "hold" water in the body, an issue usually associated with hydraulic-pressure colonics. Gravity-centered colonics also work with gravity and your body's energy to release waste, so you may actually strengthen peristalsis and your body's natural bowel moments, not weaken them.

Although it may sound counterintuitive, the more your diet improves, the more often you should get colonics. As you cleanse and wake up toxicity, colonics help remove the massive amounts of waste that have been hidden in your body. Colonics are excellent aids for helping with acne and skin eruptions as well. But if you don't change your diet first, colonics won't work as well.

If you have no access to colonics, definitely get yourself an enema kit from a drugstore or online and administer your own enemas, which you can do at home. They are not as powerful as a colonic, but are still very helpful, as they are inexpensive and you can do them regularly right in your own bathroom. Follow the directions included in the kit.

The Power of Raw Apple Cider Vinegar

Raw apple cider vinegar actually helps promote optimal digestion and encourages the growth of friendly bacteria in your body. An age-old digestive remedy calls for sipping one tablespoon of the vinegar diluted in a cup of water twenty minutes before meals, but I prefer to just include it in salad dressings. Raw apple cider vinegar is high in minerals and potassium, which help promote cellular cleansing. It has antiseptic qualities and can help cleanse your digestive tract, promoting bowel movements. Be sure that you buy a brand labeled "raw" and "unfiltered." Pasteurized apple cider vinegar does not have these healing properties.

Because of all these benefits, raw apple cider vinegar is the only acceptable vinegar you want to consume on a regular basis. You may be wondering what will become of one of your favorite salad dressing ingredients—balsamic vinegar. Balsamic vinegar is okay occasionally, but because it doesn't have the benefits of raw apple cider vinegar, it shouldn't be an everyday staple in your diet.

Magnesium-Oxygen Supplement

Consider taking a magnesium-oxygen supplement, which may have these benefits:

- Increase oxygenation in the body, which has a remarkable cleansing effect without being an irritant

- Break down, detoxify and eliminate impacted toxic waste material that has accumulated in the digestive tract

- May help balance pH in the body as it works to clean out old, acidic waste

- Enhance the body's cleansing functions, which can assist with acne and other imbalances

- Decrease bloating, gassiness and constipation

Unlike synthetic laxatives, or even harsh natural herbs with laxative properties, like senna, good-quality magnesium-oxygen supplements are non–habit forming and bolster the digestive organs' functions, making these supplements safe for regular use.

This supplement has been a huge help in my personal journey to continue cleansing myself. I have tried many different brands, as well as powders and capsules. It has been indispensible for my clients who are traveling, don't have access to colonics or simply refuse to get them. For your Beauty Detox, it's absolutely critical to consistently expel sludge from your body, in addition to eating the right foods. This supplement is designed to help you do just that. Find recommended brands and sourcing tips in the online resources section at www.kimberlysnyder.net.

EAT FRUIT ON AN EMPTY STOMACH

Fruit has the highest water content of any of the food groups, and supplies you with vital vitamins, minerals, amino acids and fatty acids. Because fruit breaks down the fastest in your system, leaving no toxic residue, it supplies you with readily available energy that can be used for immediate fuel.

The first time I talked publicly about how to eat fruit was on one of my segments for *Good Morning America.* Millions of people watched the show, and dozens of people wrote to me afterward, fascinated to know more about how to eat fruit properly. Fruit increases your vitality, delivering key vitamins, minerals and pure water into your body. However, *when* you eat fruit is key. This rule is very simple: eat fruit on an empty stomach.

You may think you're opting for the healthy choice when you go for the fruit salad for dessert, but you're just going to make digestive trouble for yourself. Fruit breaks down the quickest of all foods; it's out of the stomach in twenty to thirty minutes. If it has to sit on top of foods that take longer to digest (namely, concentrated foods like starch and protein), it will ferment and acidify the whole meal.

Fruit also digests well with leafy-green vegetables, as in the Glowing Green Smoothie, but not with starchy vegetables.

The best beauty fruits include:

Acai berries	Cranberries	Kumquats	Plums
Apples	Cucumbers	Lemons	Pomegranates
Apricots	Currants	Limes	Prunes
Avocados	Durian	Mangoes	Raisins
Bananas	Figs	Nectarines	Raspberries
Blackberries	Goji berries	Oranges	Strawberries
Blueberries	Gooseberries	Papaya	Tangerines
Cantaloupe	Grapefruit	Peaches	Tomatoes
Cherimoyas	Grapes	Pears	Watermelon
Cherries	Guava	Persimmons	
Coconut	Honeydew melon	Pineapple	

Fruit becomes a truly healthy food only when your body is cleansed enough to handle it, and when you have a good amount of healthy bacteria within to break down the fruit sugar. You have unknowingly compromised your friendly flora with antibiotics, hormonal medications (like birth control pills), preservatives, environmental pollution and many other factors. This means that, when you're first beginning your Beauty Detox, you may have an adverse reaction to fruit. If eating fruit causes nausea, burping, bloating or intense stomach upset, you may have an acidic condition in your body or sugar issues that prevent you from metabolizing fruit.

If you are more than fifty pounds overweight, come from a lifestyle of eating devitalized and processed foods, or suspect you have some kind of candidiasis or yeast imbalance in your body, remain in the Blossoming Beauty Phase (see Chapter 3) for one to three months longer than suggested, or until you have become balanced. The Blossoming Beauty Phase doesn't include sweet fruits. See more on fruit in the sugar section later in this chapter.

What Is Candidiasis and How Do I Know If I Have It?

Candidiasis, or Candida-Related Complex (CRC), is a condition that can develop when there is an overgrowth of the yeast *Candida albicans.* Many different factors cause candidiasis: taking antibiotics, birth control pills or other hormones, or eating excessive amounts of processed foods. Some symptoms include intense cravings for sugar, bread or alcoholic beverages; oppressive menstrual cramps; chronic vaginitis; chronic fungal infections of the skin or nails; long-term insomnia; chronic constipation and/or diarrhea; excessive bloating or intestinal gas; anxiety attacks; excessive emotional outbursts or crying; recurring headaches; mental spaciness; food allergies and extreme difficulty in losing weight. If these symptoms sound familiar to you, don't worry. You're not alone and there is something we can do about it!

Candidiasis is especially common in women—although many women don't even realize they have it. This yeast thrives off sugars, so you have to be very careful about what you eat until you've rid your body of candidiasis. If you even suspect that you may have it, start your Beauty Detox with the Blossoming Beauty Phase (see Chapter 3), which is sugar and gluten-free.

I have had many, many female clients who had no clue that they had candidiasis but were able to finally lose weight and get their life back after following the Blossoming Beauty Phase.

There are lab tests being developed to diagnose candidiasis and other yeast-related conditions. However, the best way to tell whether or not you have candidiasis is your history, your symptoms and how well you respond to treatment. Stay strictly in the Blossoming Beauty Phase for two weeks and see if your symptoms start to clear up. (If they improve, you've pinpointed the problem, and sticking with Blossoming Beauty for at least one to three months will usually clear it up.) However, some may need to stay in Blossoming Beauty for even longer and in extreme cases for up to a year. By closely adhering to this program, you will starve the yeast and rebalance your body once and for all. If you have had a chronic problem losing weight in the past, this rebalance could finally set you back on track for easy weight loss.

EAT HIGH-ALKALINE FOODS

All foods leave either an alkaline or an acidic residue in the bloodstream, depending on whether they contain more alkaline or more acidic minerals. Under normal circumstances, and when you're eating a diet rich in alkaline-forming foods, your body has no difficulty maintaining an optimal, slightly alkaline pH. However, when faced with an acid overload, your body has to scramble to find ways to prevent your blood pH from dropping too low, even at the expense of disrupting other tissue, organ and cellular activities in the rest of the body. With the prevalence of too much acid, the body begins to leach alkaline minerals out of the tissues to compensate. The alkaline minerals, like calcium, potassium and magnesium that you lose in the process serve many beautifying functions, such as creating strong, healthy bones and opening up detoxification pathways in your body to release aging toxins.

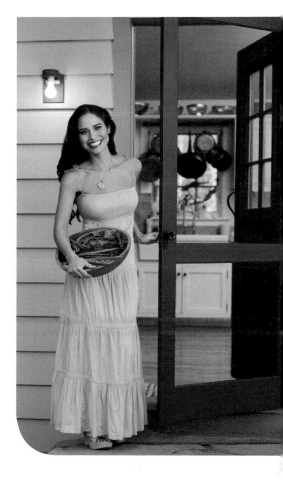

In his book *The pH Miracle,* Dr. Robert Young states, "The pH level of our internal fluids affects every cell in our bodies. The entire metabolic process depends on an alkaline environment. Chronic overacidity corrodes body tissue and, if left unchecked will interrupt all cellular activities and functions, from the beating of your heart to the neural firing of your brain. In other words, acidity interferes with life itself. It's the root of all sickness and disease." He goes on to say that "this process of acid waste breakdown and disposal could also be called 'the aging process.'"[3]

Weight loss is also much easier when your body is in an alkaline state. An acidic body tends to hold on to excess weight and makes losing weight a much bigger effort. That's because, when they're overloaded with acid, the eliminating organs, such as the lungs or the kidneys, become overwhelmed and cannot remove all the waste. This means that much of the toxic acidic waste could end up getting stored in fatty tissues all over the body. The more toxins you have in your body, the more your fat cells expand to store the toxins. Because the body is always trying to protect itself, much of the waste gets pushed away from the vital organs—which is why fat tends to collect in the usual "problem" areas, namely, under the chin, on the upper arms, across the midsection and on the hips and thighs.

An overly acidic body also greatly diminishes your beauty. Excess acidity can be a major cause of premature aging, along with premature lines and wrinkles; acne; dark under-eye circles; limp, dull or otherwise unhealthy hair; and brittle nails. These overt symptoms all start with the biochemistry of an acidic body.

THE 80:20 RATIO

The way to reach your goal to look and feel your best is to strive to eat 80 percent alkaline-forming foods and 20 percent acid-forming foods. The only foods on earth that leave a truly alkaline residue in the body are fresh, ripe fruits and vegetables and human mother's milk, which is obviously not on the menu for any of us. All other foods are, in varying degrees, acidic.

VERY ALKALINE FOODS

Greens	Ripe fruits
Other vegetables	Sprouts

VERY ACIDIC FOODS AND OTHER PRODUCTS

Alcohol	Drugs, such as antibiotics/steroids
Animal protein	Nicotine
Artificial sweeteners	Processed foods
Caffeine	Refined sugar
Dairy products	Soda

Don't get confused by the word *acidic,* which is often used to describe the taste or flavor profile of a food. For example, limes or lemons are used to add an "acid" balance to a recipe, but both digest to leave an alkaline ash in our bodies, as do most other fruits and vegetables. It is not helpful to evaluate the pH of a particular food outside the body; instead, it's the residue that foods leave when they break down inside your body that's important for your acid-alkaline balance. Dairy milk, in isolation, has an alkaline pH, but digests and leaves an extremely acidic residue in the body. Animal products also produce acidic compounds upon digestion.

Research shows the connection between increased animal protein intake and a loss of calcium in the bones, which helps neutralize the acid from consuming animal protein. In 2009, an article in the *New York Times*, titled "Exploring a Low-Acid Diet for Bone Health,"[4] asserted that "when the blood becomes even slightly too acid, alkaline calcium compounds—like calcium carbonate, the acid-neutralizer in Tums—are leached from bones to reduce the acidity." The article goes on to state, "The more protein people consume beyond the body's true needs, the more acidic their blood can become and the more alkaline compounds are needed to neutralize the acid . . . it does suggest that those at the high end of protein consumption may be better off eating less protein in general and less animal protein in particular and replacing it with more fruits and vegetables."[5]

When you focus on eating more alkaline foods, it becomes much simpler to maintain your weight and improve your health and beauty, without getting swept up in the hype of fixating over one micronutrient or another. Maintaining a high balance of foods that leave an alkaline residue in your body will naturally balance your biochemistry.

Avoid Soda

Consuming soda loads you up with lots of calories and absolutely no nutrition. But it's not just the calories we are concerned with. Soda (and that includes diet varieties, too) is also the most acid-forming of all foods. In fact, soda isn't really a food at all: it's a collection of acidic chemicals, like carbonic acid and phosphoric acid. Soda consumed regularly will demineralize your teeth and rob you of your beauty by eating up the precious minerals that create it. And don't think that you're minimizing damage by avoiding the high-calorie, regular soda: an eight-year study of collected data revealed that your risk of becoming overweight is 32.8 percent if you drink one to two cans of soda a day, but if you drink one or two cans of diet soda a day instead, your risk goes up to 54.5 percent.[6] (See more on the artificial sweeteners contained in diet sodas later in this chapter.)

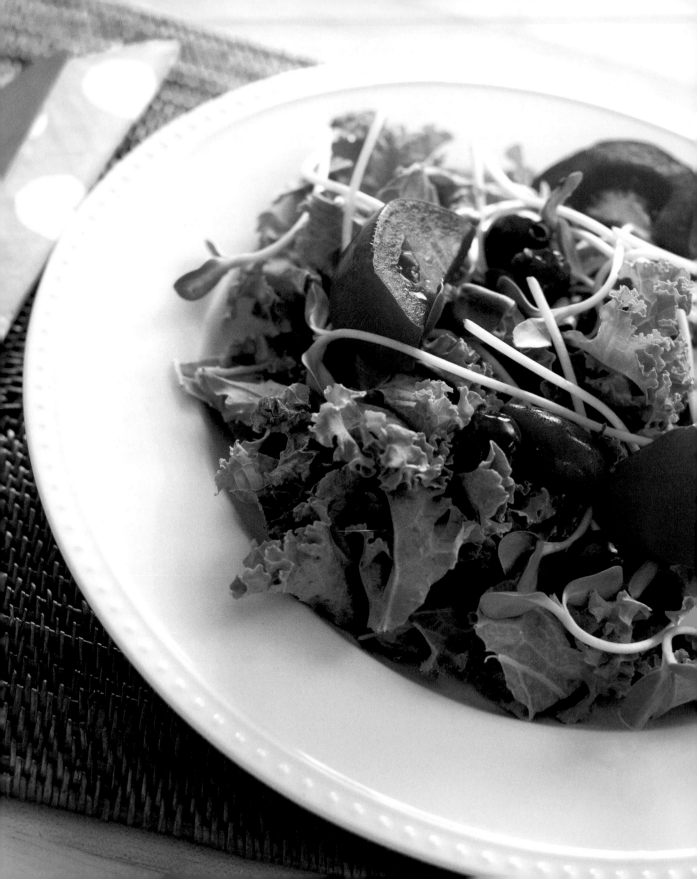

EAT ALKALINE FIRST

At each meal, no matter what the whole meal will entail, begin by putting an alkaline food first in the body—the best choices include some Glowing Green Smoothie (I sometimes drink more of it while cooking dinner), raw vegetables or salad. Besides ensuring that you consistently load up on raw plant enzymes, practicing this rule will ensure that you get alkaline, water-containing foods in the body at every meal and increase the overall percentage of these foods in your diet.

Do you notice something that these alkaline foods have in common? They contain a great deal of fiber. Fiber acts as a cushion to help slow down glucose absorption in the bloodstream and prevents your blood sugar levels from becoming elevated and erratic. Fiber also fills you up and helps diminish your physiological cravings. It's an easy, delicious way to control portion sizes naturally. When you fill up first with fresh, natural foods, you can eat in abundance and never feel deprived, since these foods have so much filling fiber and contain so many nutrients. Plus, it's easy to have a salad at the start of lunch and dinner at a restaurant or when preparing meals at home.

Fiber also helps keep your digestive tract functioning optimally and keeps you regular, which is critical for your ongoing cleansing efforts. It helps to consistently remove waste from the body. A report published in the *Journal of the National Cancer Institute* suggested that if one's daily fiber intake was increased by thirteen grams, the risk of colon cancer would decrease by 31 percent.[7] The solution is not to add an isolated fiber supplement, like Metamucil, to a diet filled with foods sorely lacking in crucial dietary fiber. Americans spend $725 million a year on laxatives alone.[8] Something is clearly wrong. Instead, focus on increasing your percentage of high-fiber foods, aka plant foods. There is no fiber—repeat, none!—in animal products. Average Americans get only about eight to fourteen grams of fiber a day in their diet. Eating Beauty Detox foods, you will get much more—upwards of forty grams or more of fiber.[9] Sixteen ounces of the Glowing Green Smoothie alone contains over 13 grams of fiber!

It's important to plan ahead. For example, if you're going to a Chinese restaurant for lunch with your coworkers and you know you may have a hard time finding raw vegetables there, keep some crudités or baby spinach leaves on hand, and eat them within the hour before lunch. When I travel and I know I will be eating less than optimally, I always carry some celery or carrot sticks that I can eat to make sure I have alkaline food before a potentially highly acidic meal.

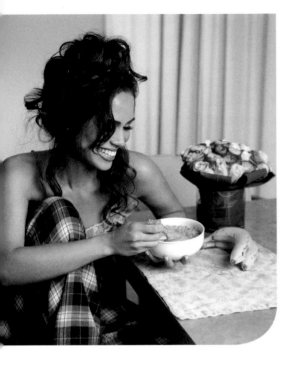

EAT BEAUTIFUL CARBOHYDRATES AND STARCHES

Carbohydrates, also known as starches or sugars, are a macronutrient that provides you with energy. You may be uneasy about consuming too many starches because you're accustomed to counting calories and carbs. But diets like that are about restriction, and often leave you feeling unsatisfied, or thinking about food way too much. The most slender cultures in the world, those across Asia, Africa and South America, eat low-fat, vegetable- and starch-based diets.

The goal of the Beauty Detox program is to free up Beauty Energy, speed up digestion and clean out sludge from your system, not tally up numbers on your calculator. The high-quality, complex carbs you'll be eating on the plan help accomplish all those things and are easily digestible. This means that carbs, in the form of refined, processed starch and processed or artificial sugars, are completely off your menu.

THE KEY TO EATING CARBS

There are three types of carbohydrates: complex, simple and fiber. Complex carbohydrates, also known as starches, include whole, unrefined grains and fiber-rich starches like root vegetables. Simple carbohydrates, also known as sugars, provide the body with fast energy; they include all refined starches and sugars, as well as fruits. Fiber is a kind of complex carbohydrate that is undigested by your body. The key to carbohydrates is to eat the correct high-quality forms.

Natural grain kernels contain the bran, endosperm and germ. Refined carbohydrates—including white-flour breads, pastas and pastries, as well as white rice, many breakfast cereals, and most packaged cookies, snacks and baked goods—have been processed to remove the bran and germ. This refinement process removes not only the fiber but also many of the minerals, vitamins and nutrients—in other words, all the good stuff from the grain. Refined carbohydrates steal your energy and make you feel tired and lazy.

BEAUTY GRAINS

The best Beauty Detox grains are millet, quinoa (pronounced KEEN-wah), amaranth and buckwheat. These grains are gluten-free and all, except for buckwheat, also known as kasha (which leaves a slightly acid-forming residue), digest to leave an alkaline residue in the body. Brown rice is also an acceptable option. Although you want to fill up on veggies first to control portion size, these grains add important fiber and denseness to a meal, can be prepared in delicious low-fat ways and help stop cravings for refined carbs, like breads and pastries.

Even though you may not have ever eaten these grains in the past, they are generally easy to find. In fact, you'll find that it's easy enough to swap these grains for your current starch staples, like white rice and pasta. Quinoa is sold at stores like Trader Joe's and is regularly stocked in your local grocery store. They are inexpensive (a pound of millet is around $2 or $3), easy to cook and prepare, and make delicious accompaniments to veggies and salads. Products made from these grains are also available, including millet bread, millet cereal, kasha cereal, quinoa crackers, quinoa pasta, quinoa flakes and cream of buckwheat cereal. When you switch to these grains and grain products, you will not miss anything—that is, except for the excess pounds.

It's important to soak grains at least eight hours, and preferably overnight. This will help deactivate the enzyme inhibitors that coat all grains (and beans) and will make them even easier to digest. Get in the habit of planning ahead. Soak some quinoa or millet the night before, and make enough to last you for a couple of days or to pack for lunch.

The reality is that sometimes you might have trouble finding certain products, like millet bread, when you're traveling or eating out. (What? You mean Barnacle Billy's doesn't offer millet bread?) The key in these situations is to do your best. Rice is a better option than wheat, and brown rice is a better choice than refined white rice. Brown rice flour is terrific for gluten-free baking, as you'll see in Part III. Anytime you eat a grain or starch product, and especially when you eat these less than ideal grain or starch products, take a digestive enzyme to help them digest better. And remember, it's the norm, not the occasional exceptions to the rule, that counts.

AVOID GLUTEN FOR BETTER BEAUTY

Contrary to popular belief, whole-wheat bread, bagels, crackers and other products are not so beautiful for the body. Although wheat is an ancient crop, the wheat farmed today is hardly what wheat once was in its original form. Today, wheat is grown in mineral-depleted soil and is heavily sprayed with pesticides and other chemicals. You want to reduce all exposure to these potentially beauty-squashing toxic chemicals, which find their way into your body through the wheat and wheat-based products you eat. Moreover, in addition to containing these toxic pesticides, wheat is stored for long periods in silos and may often be contaminated to varying degrees with molds and fungi, which steal your Beauty Energy.

Wheat is one of the eight most common foods that account for about 90 percent of all allergic reactions in the United States. The others are milk, eggs, peanuts, tree nuts (like cashews), fish, shellfish and soy.[10] What makes wheat so allergenic is the gluten in it, which is its primary protein. Gluten, which is also present in rye, farro and barley, may cause toxic reactions that trigger your immune system and may cause inflammation of the intestinal tract. Many people may be sensitive to gluten because of overexposure (a common way to develop food allergies), as wheat is snuck into many processed foods.

You may have an intolerance to gluten and may not even be aware of it or experience any overt symptoms. James Braly, M.D., and Ron Hoggan, M.A., coauthors of the book *Dangerous Grains: Why Gluten Cereal Grains May Be Hazardous to Your Health,* claim that gluten intolerance is a factor not only in celiac disease (an autoimmune disease in which the lining of the small intestine is damaged by the consumption of wheat and, as a result, cannot process gluten) but also in many autoimmune disorders and neurological and psychiatric conditions, including rheumatoid arthritis, hyperthyroidism and liver disease.[11]

Eliminating highly and commonly allergenic foods, such as gluten, from your diet may help improve your overall health, help eliminate sugar and carb cravings, help stabilize your mood and help you lose weight. You may not feel results immediately when you go gluten-free, because it can take some time for any inflammation to decrease. But over time, you'll notice the positive difference.

I have seen these positive effects in many of my clients, but I've also experienced them for myself. Since cutting out gluten, I have noticed that my energy level has improved and my weight has stabilized—and I don't crave bread anymore the way I used to.

To achieve your highest level of beauty, work toward cutting out all wheat products, including cereals, pastries, pastas, breads, pretzels, cookies, seitan (pure gluten), bagels and the like. On the other hand, also avoid all the gluten-free products cropping up that are made of mostly cheap, low-nutrient ingredients, such as corn or potato flour. Don't panic! I know this seems like a long list of foods to give up, and it may seem scary, but it's not. This doesn't mean you'll never eat a piece of bread again for the rest of your life. You'll just replace wheat and wheat products with much higher-quality grains. When you have a break from wheat and notice how much better you feel and look, you'll have a lot of motivation to keep avoiding it and sticking to the better replacements.

Your best beauty choices include:

Amaranth	Quinoa
Buckwheat (also called kasha)	Soba noodles (made of buckwheat)
Millet	Starchy vegetables (winter squash, yams, sweet potatoes, etc.)

Your next-best beauty choices include:

Beans, all varieties (more info on beans on page 60)	Chickpeas
Black-eyed peas	Gluten-free crackers, pastas and other foods
Brown or wild rice	Lentils

Your worst beauty choices—avoid these!—include:

Gluten-free products made of mainly corn or potato flour	Rye and barley
	Wheat and wheat products
Processed and refined starches and sugars	White rice

STARCHY VEGETABLES: A BEAUTIFUL CHOICE

Starchy vegetables are an excellent addition to a meal. They taste great and satisfy your hunger. There are so many incredible starchy vegetables and tubers out there. Among the best are red-jacket potatoes, all varieties of squash, and sweet potatoes and yams. Have fun looking into varieties that you don't already know about. There's yucca, spaghetti squash, acorn squash, kabocha squash, butternut squash and many more. The best way to eat these starchy vegetables is to cook them well; in this case they digest better and taste better, too. Yams, winter squash and sweet potatoes can be thoroughly baked at high temperatures. Check out Beauty Detox recipes containing squash and other starchy beauty vegetables in Part III.

AVOID SUGARS

In addition to refined starches like white flour, you have to watch out for refined sugars, like agave, sucrose, lactose, white sugar, brown sugar, molasses, fruit juice concentrates and high-fructose corn syrup. Refined sugar is one of the most toxic foods you can eat: it causes extreme energy fluctuations, intense cravings and feelings of depression, anger and anxiety.

Studies have shown sugar to be more addictive than cocaine,[12] so it's no wonder that sugar is one of the primary cravings that people experience. Let's look at the numbers:

The more sugar you eat, the more your taste buds become conditioned to it, and the more you need to feel satisfied.[13] It even sounds like a drug!

How Sugar Destroys Your Beauty

Let's discuss some specific ways that sugar destroys your beauty:

- ⊙ **Sugar gives you wrinkles.** Although sugar is causing damage to organs on the inside of your body, it's also causing you to look older.[14] The way sugar binds with proteins and fats causes aging, cellular free-radical damage as well as stiffening the collagen in your skin, making it inflexible and creating wrinkles.[15] Goodbye youthful, supple skin. You'll find more information on the research on page 52.

- ⊙ **Sugar makes you move more stiffly.** Compare the ease with which a teenager walks down the street with, say, someone with creaky joints and a stooped back in his or her eighties. If you can't move fluidly, no matter what your chronological age, you'll look older. Sugar interacts with proteins in your body to create sticky bonds; interferes with the production of new collagen throughout the entire body, including the joints; and can trigger arthritis and tissue damage.

- ⊙ **Sugar makes you fat.** Sugar makes your body insensitive to the hormones insulin and leptin (which are key for helping to reduce hunger), and this insensitivity can lead to weight gain and diabetes. Over time and with overexposure, your body can no longer hear the messages telling it to stop eating and burn fat—so it remains hungry and stores more fat. Leptin resistance also causes an increase in visceral fat, sending you on a vicious cycle of hunger, fat storage and an increased risk of heart disease and diabetes, among other ills. Excess sugar may disrupt the hormones signaling your body to build muscle.

- ◉ **Sugar steals your beauty nutrients.** Sugar upsets the mineral relationships in your body, causes chromium and copper deficiencies, and interferes with absorption of calcium and magnesium.[16] It can also leach out the important beauty vitamin, vitamin E.[17]

- ◉ **Sugar reduces the function of enzymes,** which you need for energy.[18]

- ◉ **Sugar taxes your adrenals,**[19] leading to physical beauty issues, like dark under-eye circles.

- ◉ **Sugar hinders your ongoing cleansing.** Sugar can be constipating,[20] and encourages bad intestinal bacteria, yeasts and fungi to flourish, which can overwhelm the digestive tract and lead to indigestion and constipation.[21]

In addition, sugar is grating to your nerves and causes surges of adrenaline and other hormone fluctuations, which may be irritating to the brain. Try cutting your sugar habit down, and watch your headaches diminish.

The Glycemic Index: Not the Be-All and End-All

Over the past few decades, the glycemic index (GI) has become a bit of a buzzword. The GI is a measure of the effect of a particular food on your blood sugar.

But the GI is not the only deciding factor on whether a food is healthy or not. Fructose has a low GI ranking, since it doesn't stimulate surges of insulin to be released from the pancreas in the way that glucose (another type of sugar molecule) does. But high levels of fructose especially in refined liquid, fiberless forms, such as high-fructose corn syrup, is associated with serious health issues, such as insulin resistance, cardiovascular complications, elevated blood fats and obesity,[22] and should be avoided.

Furthermore, certain foods, like bananas, papayas, apricots and carrots, have a higher GI number, but they are still natural, healthy foods. You don't want to eat a diet loaded with all high-glycemic foods, but some nutrient-dense foods that have a higher GI, such as some fruits and vegetables, are healthy and have lots of plant fiber. A diet loaded with dietary fiber that includes fruits, vegetables and certain natural, unrefined whole-grain carbohydrates will help stabilize blood sugar levels. In fact, some researchers believe that it's the presence or lack of plant fiber that is the most reliable indicator of blood glucose control.[23] The bottom line is this: you will reach your ultimate health and beauty goals by eating a diet filled with nutrient- and fiber-rich foods in their natural, unrefined and unprocessed state.

"Should I Avoid Fruit Because of the Sugar?"

What about fruit?, you may ask yourself. *Does fruit have too much sugar?* While it is true that fruit contains natural sugars, whole fruit comes in a complete nutritional package along with fiber. Eating fruit is entirely different than consuming refined sugars, or agave or high-fructose corn syrup—two liquid products extremely high in fructose—that contain no fiber and are not whole foods, and allow you to consume large amounts in one sitting. Fruit also contains high levels of antioxidants and vitamin C, which are said to help neutralize the effects of the natural fructose and other sugars it contains.[24]

The cleaner your body becomes, the better it can handle fruit, allowing you to then truly realize its powerful cleansing abilities. If you've eaten a compromised diet in the past or have a great deal of slow-digesting fat and/or protein in your diet, you may not handle fruit well and may feel bloated or experience other detrimental affects from eating it. If you have candidiasis (see more on page 38), all fruit except non-sweet fruit should be avoided for a period. Those with diabetes and other specific health conditions should also carefully monitor fruit intake. Straight fruit juice with its fiber stripped is never recommended.

However, as your health builds over time, fruit is not only incredibly beautifying, but will be a weight loss aid. It digests cleanly and quickly, contains no fat, and is extremely alkaline, which will help balance your pH and dissolve acids and toxins from the body, which may contribute to stored weight in your body.

During the first few years of improving my diet I didn't eat too much fruit. Now that my diet is properly balanced and low in fat, I eat a great deal of whole fruit (particularly pineapple and papaya), and thrive. My body looks more toned from increased cleansing, and my energy soars. I stay slim, and my skin glows.

Sugars to Avoid

It's absolutely critical to eliminate sodas, refined starches and all straight fruit juices (orange juice, apple juice and so on)—starting right now. If beauty and health are of any real concern to you, go cold turkey on this. There are so many good alternatives, so there really is no excuse not to.

In addition, avoid sugar in all its sneaky forms. Here are some of the names sugar goes by:

Agave	Crystalline fructose	Invert sugar	Muscovato
Barley malt syrup	Dextrose	Malt	Succanat
Brown rice syrup	Evaporated cane juice	Malt syrup	Sucrose
Corn sweeteners	Fructose	Maltodextrin	Turbinado sugar
Corn syrup	High-fructose corn syrup	Maltose	

Two of these—high-fructose corn syrup and agave—have been the subject of particularly distressing studies:

- **High-fructose corn syrup:** I'm always frustrated when I see ads proclaiming high-fructose corn syrup as a safe and natural sweetener. In fact, it is a cheap and highly processed sweetener derived from corn. High-fructose corn syrup (HFCS) began replacing corn sugar in processed foods, such as soft drinks, breakfast cereals, cookies and many other baked goods, in the 1980s, parallel to the rise of obesity. Due to its cheap production costs, manufacturers are using more of it and getting more people hooked on supersized portions of soft drinks and sweet junk food, while still making big profits. A study that appeared in the June 2008 issue of the *Journal of Nutrition,* called "Dietary Sugars Stimulate Fatty Acid Synthesis in Adults," concluded that fructose gets converted into fat more quickly than glucose,[25] making HFCS particularly fattening.

A recent study out of Princeton University and published in *Pharmacology Biochemistry and Behavior* found that high-fructose corn syrup causes considerably more weight gain than table sugar. Princeton professor Bart Hoebel, who specializes in the neuroscience of appetite, weight and sugar addiction, one of the study's authors, explained: "Some people have claimed that high-fructose corn syrup is no different than other sweeteners when it comes to weight gain and obesity, but our results make it clear that this just isn't true, at least under the conditions of our tests. When rats are drinking high-fructose corn syrup at levels well below those in soda pop, they're becoming obese—every single one, across the board. Even when rats are fed a high-fat diet, you don't see this; they don't all gain extra weight."[26]

◉ **Agave:** Also called agave syrup and agave nectar, this sweetener is becoming increasingly popular as "healthy" and "low glycemic." It is *not* a healthy sweetener choice, and, as you'll soon learn, agave can seriously age your skin. Today it's found not only in health food stores but even in mainstream grocery stores, as well as in energy bars, drinks, other food products and health and raw food recipes. Years ago, I used to use and promote it myself. But now that I have learned more about it and how it's processed, I have cut it out of my diet altogether, and it is a mission of mine to educate others as much as possible to avoid agave completely as well, so they can avoid damaging their health and beauty. It's true that agave nectar is low on the glycemic index, but it also has a fructose content of upwards of an alarming 90 percent, which is much higher than even high-fructose corn syrup, which averages about 55 percent fructose. As Dr. Ingrid Kohlstadt, a fellow of the American College of Nutrition and an associate faculty member at the Johns Hopkins School of Public Health, points out, "Agave is almost all fructose, a highly processed sugar with great marketing."[27]

Fructose also has potential to greatly increase the aging of your skin through oxidative damage. Advanced glycation end products (AGEs) are created when sugars react with proteins in the body, damaging collagen by "cross-linking" or having the individual collagen fibers glue or stick together. This cross-linking forms little scars in the collagen that, over time, can become deeper and deeper and lead to visible wrinkles. Now there's a word we all know the meaning of. In a lab study, researchers found that the group of rats given fructose had more cross-linking changes in the collagen of their skin than the rats that were fed glucose.[28] In fact, Richard J. Johnson, M.D., writes in his book *The Sugar Fix: The High-Fructose Fallout That Is Making You Fat and Sick,* that some research suggests that fructose is up to ten times more efficient than glucose in producing AGEs.[29] Yes, you read it right. Ten times!

Agave is a big no-no that must be avoided by all who want to preserve youthful skin. Agave syrup, or agave nectar, is not a whole food found in nature. Instead, it usually has to undergo extensive processing to arrive at that sweet liquid syrup form, and this may involve many chemicals and/or heating processes, even if the agave syrup is labeled "raw."[30] Strictly avoid foods and restaurant dishes (salad dressings, desserts, etc.) that include agave in their ingredients list.

Stevia and Other Sweet Choices

One of the best sweeteners to use is stevia, which you can buy in a powdered or a concentrated liquid form. Stevia is a natural herb that has been used for hundreds of years in South America and grows naturally in parts of Paraguay and Brazil. It's widely available in the marketplace today. It is my go-to sweetener for everything from smoothies to baking (see Part III). Some people find it bitter at first, but your taste buds adapt. I used to think that, too, but now I don't notice any bitterness at all. Different stevia brands have different tastes, so don't give up if one brand turned you off. Please visit the online resources section of www.kimberlysnyder.net for stevia brands I recommend.

Here is a list of a few other sweetener choices that should be used in strict moderation:

- Raw coconut nectar is my first liquid sweetener choice. When the coconut tree is tapped, it produces a naturally sweet nectar that comes from the coconut blossoms. It is nutrient-rich, containing seventeen amino acids, minerals, vitamin C and B vitamins. Its fructose content is only about 10 percent, compared to upwards of 90 percent in agave. It doesn't have a coconut taste, and you can find it pretty commonly now in the sweetener section of health food markets or online.

- Small amounts of dried fruit, such as figs and dates, can be used as sweeteners when blended in certain recipes. Eating these foods on their own is best enjoyed by athletes and very active people, as they are sugar and calorically dense foods.

- Raw honey contains fructose, but it's a whole, natural food (although not vegan). Be sure to purchase only raw honey that is organic, and, if possible, purchase locally from a beekeeper who uses ethical practices.

- Organic, pure maple syrup is another choice when you need a liquid sweetener. It's not raw, because it undergoes heat processing, and it's made up of sucrose, but it doesn't require as much processing as agave and artificial sweeteners, and is a much better choice than those.

- Xylitol, a low-glycemic substitute that is actually a sugar alcohol naturally occurring in the fibers of fruits and vegetables, is also an acceptable option. Xylitol is contained in some chewing gums, and it may help reduce cavity-causing bacteria in teeth. Be moderate in your xylitol consumption, however; consuming too much may lead to bloating, gassiness and diarrhea.

- Erythritol is another sugar alcohol naturally occurring in fruits and other foods. It has zero calories and is only partially absorbed in the small intestine.

Say No to Splenda

Although they have all been approved and declared "safe" for human consumption, there is a lot of controversy and potential health risks associated with artificial sweeteners, which include aspartame (Equal and NutraSweet), saccharin (Sweet 'N Low) and sucralose (Splenda).

Let's start with aspartame, also known as NutraSweet and Equal. Aspartame is an excitotoxin, which is a toxic substance that in high concentrations may stimulate nerve cells so much that they are damaged or killed. It's composed of aspartic acid, methyl ester (which breaks down to formaldehyde and formic acid) and phenylalanine. Those are scary words, right? They point to one thing: that they are acid-forming in the body.

Think aspartame can help you lose weight? Guess again. Despite the fact that it has zero calories, studies have shown that aspartame can actually induce weight gain. Some researchers believe that two of the main ingredients in aspartame—phenylalanine and aspartic acid—stimulate the release of insulin and interfere with normal communication with the hormone leptin, promoting fat storage in your body.[31]

Phenylalanine is an essential amino acid, but unnaturally high, isolated amounts of it can act as a neurotoxin, overexciting neurons in the brain. Aspartame contains high levels of isolated phenylalanine. One study showed that when people ingest a large amount of phenylalanine, it can drive down the levels of serotonin,[32] which is the neurotransmitter that tells you when you're full. A low level of serotonin can also bring on food cravings.

Saccharin, aka Sweet 'N Low, is no better in this regard. A study at Purdue University's Ingestive Behavior Research Center concluded that consuming foods sweetened with saccharin leads to greater weight gain and body fat than eating the same foods sweetened with sugar.[33]

What about the new, popular sweetener sucralose, aka Splenda? Researchers from the Duke University Medical Center published a study in the *Journal of Toxicology and Environmental Health* showing that sucralose lowered good bacteria in the intestines by 50 percent and contributed to an increase in body weight in lab studies.[34] The best bet is to avoid all these artificial sweeteners and all products that contain them: they have too many potential health risks. The better choice for a calorie-free sweetener is stevia.

EAT MORE PLANT PROTEIN

Protein is probably the most poorly understood category of foods there is. And no wonder, given that an ever-growing number of confusing studies and statistics are put out about protein. And although you may have tried cutting out carb grams or fat grams during different dieting fads over the last few decades, I'll bet you have never heard it be suggested that you cut back on the highly touted macronutrient called protein. In fact, you are led to believe that you can never consume too much protein. Popular wisdom is that protein helps you lose weight and gives you muscle tone, so we're told to cut back on calories, carbs, fat grams, yes, but never protein. Does this sound familiar?

One of the first things a vegetarian is asked is, "Where do you get your protein?" This highlights the misconception that only meat and animal products contain protein, and that if you don't eat meat, you're at risk for protein deficiency. I admit that I used to wonder whether I was getting enough protein when I stopped eating animal products altogether. I used to supplement my diet with protein powders daily, and portioned out a certain amount of nuts to eat every day. But I stopped these practices years ago. I now know that I get more than enough protein from my plant-based diet, without trying to supplement protein. I feel better than ever, and my body is more toned than it has ever been.

Let's back up for a minute to get a wider view of this protein issue. Your body doesn't use protein per se. It uses amino acids. Many of the largest, most muscular animals on earth—gorillas, wild horses, hippos, rhinos—are vegetarians. They efficiently build up the protein and muscles in their body from the amino acids in the greens they eat. The false idea of having to eat animal protein to build muscle has long been held up in society. But today, as more information becomes available on the benefits of a plant-based diet, more people (even athletes) are choosing not to eat animal protein, and are becoming healthier and performing better.

There are twenty-three different amino acids, fourteen that the body manufactures on its own and nine that cannot be manufactured by the body and must come from diet alone. When a food contains all nine of these amino acids—known as the essential amino acids—it's called a complete protein. These nine essential amino acids (phenylalanine, valine, lysine, leucine, isoleucine, tryptophan, threonine, histidine and methionine) are found in abundance in fruits, vegetables, seeds, sprouts and nuts. Some examples of great plant-based food sources of amino acids are these:

Asparagus	Cabbage	Nuts and seeds (all of them)
Broccoli	Cauliflower	Spinach
Brussels sprouts	Kale	Sprouts

By consuming a wide variety of foods from these various plant groups, you will receive the essential nine amino acids in abundance. Furthermore, you don't need to carefully combine foods to get all nine essential amino acids at each meal. A bestselling book in the 1960s called *Diet for a Small Planet* popularized the idea of "protein combining." But in 1981 the author herself, Frances Moore Lappé, rewrote the book to reflect the fact that her previous theories of protein combining had been misinformed. Your body stores and releases the amino acids needed over a twenty-four-hour period to supplement your daily amino acid intake and ensure you get all the amino acids you need.[35] The body also has an amino acid pool and recycles proteins on a regular basis. Keep in mind that amino acids are delicate entities. Most animal protein is cooked, which can denature the amino acids and make them largely unavailable for your body's use.[36] The Max Planck Institute for Nutritional Research in Germany discovered that cooking destroys about 50 percent of the bioavailability of protein for humans.[37]

The American Dietetic Association states that "plant protein can meet protein requirements when a variety of plant foods is consumed" and "research indicates that an assortment of plant foods eaten over the course of a day can provide all essential amino acids and ensure adequate nitrogen retention and use in healthy adults; thus, complementary proteins don't need to be consumed at the same meal."[38]

When you're eating real plant food—greens, other veggies, sprouts, fruit, seeds and nuts—in abundance, protein deficiency is not a problem. And as I stated in Chapter 1, if you are consuming an adequate amount of daily calories, it is virtually impossible for you to be deficient in protein.

GREENS AND OTHER VEGETABLES

Greens are packed with easily assimilated amino acids. Besides the Glowing Green drinks (see Chapter 1), strive to eat vibrant, raw salads made of leafy greens every day. When you compare calories to protein content, per one hundred calories, broccoli has 11.2 grams of protein, as compared with steak, which has only 5.4 grams. Romaine lettuce has 11.6 grams of protein per one hundred calories.[39] Calorie for calorie, plant food has almost twice as much protein as meat. Sure you have to eat a greater volume of plant food, but that is a good thing—the more plant foods you eat, the more nutrients and fiber you'll get. Not so with animal protein.

NUTS AND SEEDS

Raw nuts and seeds are a great source of protein. Nuts are a highly concentrated and calorically dense food, so you need to balance them by making sure you eat some greens and raw veggies before them and along with them, and never eat them with animal products. One to two ounces is the maximum daily amount. If you are an active person or an athlete, or you're trying to gain or maintain weight, the portion size can be adjusted slightly higher.

The best beauty nuts and seeds include:

Almonds	Filberts	Hemp seeds	Pumpkin seeds	Walnuts
Brazil nuts	Flaxseeds	Pecans	Sesame seeds	
Chia seeds	Hazelnuts	Pine nuts	Sunflower seeds	

Here are a few more tips:

- **Nuts and seeds must always be eaten raw.** Roasting alters some of the nuts' beneficial qualities, and commercially packaged seeds and nuts are sometimes cooked in hydrogenated oils, which are full of unhealthy trans fats, and salted.

- **Always soak nuts and seeds in water before eating them.** Nuts and seeds have inhibitor enzymes on their surface to protect them from germinating until it's safe to do so. Soaking helps deactivate the inhibitor enzymes so that the nutrients are more readily available. Soaking also activates beneficial enzymes and helps convert many of the stored nutrients from a dormant to an active and available state. If you don't soak your raw nuts and seeds, they will be more acid-forming in the body. (Note that roasted nuts and seeds cannot be soaked.) To soak, place the nuts or seeds in a container and cover them with one to two inches of water. The harder the consistency of a nut or seed, the longer you need to soak it. For instance, hard nuts, such as almonds, require at least twenty-four hours; medium-density nuts, such as walnuts or Brazil nuts, require around six hours; and soft nuts, such as pine nuts and macadamia nuts, require only two hours or less. Soak seeds like sunflower and pumpkin seeds overnight. The nuts and seeds will plump up as they absorb the water. If you're soaking nuts or seeds overnight, you should rinse them off before using them. They can stay totally submerged in water for up to two days in the fridge. I often throw a bunch of different nuts into a bowl and let them soak overnight to save time. If you want the nuts to be totally dry for a certain recipe or to snack on, you can dehydrate them after soaking. A dehydrator is basically a low-temperature mini-oven, which dries foods over long periods at low temperatures that preserve foods' natural enzymes.

- **Eat cashews in strict moderation or avoid them altogether.** Cashews are more susceptible to various potentially toxic molds (which may be why so many people are allergic to them). They are almost always steamed to remove their tough outer shell, so technically they are rarely truly raw, and therefore are not sproutable and shouldn't be soaked. Although I use them occasionally in some recipes that should be eaten in moderation, like dessert treats, they are certainly not a daily food. Don't worry, though. There are lots of other healthy nuts to choose from instead.

- **Stick to the one-or-two-ounce-a-day maximum amount.** Nuts have a lot of healthful qualities, but they're dense and contain fairly high amounts of fat, albeit "healthy" fat.

I see a lot of raw foodists gain a lot of weight and become sluggish because they attempt to replace the cooked food in their diet with copious amounts of nuts (*but it's raw!* they say), which in large portion sizes are acid-forming and fattening. Beware of "gourmet" raw food dishes that by eating, you may unknowingly consume an alarming amount of nuts. It's better to incoporate low-fat, gluten-free options, such as quinoa or millet, instead of overdoing the nuts.

Pass on Peanuts

Peanuts are technically a legume, although most people think of them as a nut. I purposely left peanuts off the list of recommended legumes or nuts, because they are prone to mold and fungi. This may be why so many people have allergic reactions to them. Nonorganic peanuts are also among the most pesticide-saturated foods in the Western diet. A study in 1993 found that there were twenty-four different types of fungi that colonized inside peanuts, even after sterilizing their exterior.[40] A toxic mold called aflatoxin tends to contaminate peanuts, as demonstrated in studies in England[41] and at MIT.[42] In 1988 the International Agency for Research on Cancer (IARC) placed aflatoxin B_1 on the list of human carcinogens, and aflatoxin is considered a potent chemical carcinogen twenty times more toxic than DDT. A number of epidemiological studies were done in Asia and Africa that demonstrated a positive association between dietary aflatoxins and liver cell cancer.[43]

Why risk eating mold? I recommend sticking to organic, raw almond butter and other varieties of nut butters, and avoiding peanuts altogether.

CHLORELLA AND SPIRULINA

Chlorella, a form of green algae, is about 65 percent protein, which means there are about fifteen grams of protein in one tablespoon. Spirulina, a blue-green algae, is about 60 percent protein, but since it's less dense, you would have to consume larger quantities of it to get the same amount of protein as in chlorella. Spirulina is also rich in gamma-linolenic acid (GLA), B vitamins, omega-3 fatty acids and enzymes. Both bring you an inner glow and are discussed further in Chapter 8.

Spirulina and chlorella are both algaes that contain all the essential amino acids and are high in chlorophyll. Both of these algaes are considered a tonic and rejuvenator of the body. They are great to take in powdered or pill form when traveling, when fresh greens are not readily available. They can be helpful in warding off energy slumps and, thanks to their high protein content, they are useful for active athletes.[44] If you're an athlete or are on the go, I recommend taking chlorella tablets after a workout or keeping them in your purse or carry-on bag. Chewing these tablets will temporarily satisfy your hunger and provide you with pure protein and necessary minerals.

LEGUMES AND BEANS

Legumes and beans are an inexpensive protein source that is great for the transitional diet, especially during the Blossoming Beauty Phase (see Chapter 3), and for anyone switching to a vegetarian diet. They have favorable qualities, such as a high protein content and an abundance of certain minerals, vitamins and phytonutrients. But unless you consume the raw sprouted varieties instead of the fully cooked ones, I put legumes and beans in fourth place, after greens and other vegetables, nuts and seeds, and spirulina and chlorella.

Why? First of all, legumes are nature's "oops," in that they contain both protein and starch. Because they incorporate both classes of food, they are difficult to digest—which is exactly why they cause bloating, burping, flatulence, abdominal discomfort and a feeling of heaviness. Still, legumes and beans are great for the transition diet and are okay when enjoyed occasionally, especially when soaked overnight to help you digest them better if you are preparing them yourself. If you're in a tight time jam, consider cooking beans in bulk and freezing some. Canned beans should generally be avoided, as cans often contain bisphenol A (BPA) and other toxins, which can leach into foods. Cartons of pre-cooked beans are now available at certain health food stores, and sit next to the canned beans on the shelf, and may be a safer option. The following is a list of some best beauty legumes and beans, but there are many other varieties.

Adzuki beans	Great northern beans	Lima beans
Black beans	Green peas	Mung beans
Black-eyed peas	Kidney beans	Navy beans
Garbanzo beans (chickpeas)	Lentils	Pinto beans

AVOID (MOST) SOY PRODUCTS

Chances are, in one form or another, you've heard that soy is a "miracle" food that is a great alternative protein source. The growing soy industry would love to have you believe that. But soy may not be the miracle health food we have all been led to believe it is.

You may be scratching your head and wondering why you've heard of healthy Asian cultures that consume soy. The truth is that Asians don't consume the enormous amount of soy that Americans consume, but rather use soy as a side dish to rice, vegetables and small quantities of fish and meat. Furthermore, Asians don't consume all the highly processed soy protein isolates and concentrates that are most popular in the United States today.

Soy protein isolates are common ingredients in protein powders and packaged food and energy bars. These isolates undergo extensive heat processing in large commercial labs, processing that usually includes acid-washing in aluminum tanks and spray-drying at high temperatures. To produce textured vegetable protein (TVP), a common ingredient found in processed vegetarian food, high-temperature processing is also necessary.

Let's explore some of the major problems with soy:

⊙ **Soy is a top allergenic food, and the majority of soy in the United States is genetically engineered.**[45] Genetic engineering greatly alters the nutrient chemistry in certain foods. You want to avoid genetically modified organisms (GMOs). Genetically engineered soy is reported to have 29 percent less choline, a mineral needed for the development of your nervous system, and 200 percent more lectin, which is associated with food sensitivities.[46] This could be why soy is now one of the top ten allergenic foods in America.

⊙ **Soy contains trypsin inhibitors.** Trypsin is an enzyme that is needed to digest and assimilate protein properly. Trypsin inhibitors may reduce protein digestion and amino acid uptake.[47]

⊙ **Soy depresses your thyroid function.** Soy also contains isoflavones, which are substances that have been shown to depress thyroid function.[48] The thyroid controls metabolism, among other essential processes in the body, and slowing it down contributes to weight gain. One study showed that genistein in soy foods can cause irreversible damage to enzymes that synthesize thyroid hormones.[49]

ABC's *20/20* did an investigative report in June 2000 on the health claims of soy.[50] As part of the investigation, *20/20* cited a letter by Daniel Doerge and Daniel Sheehan, two of the Food and Drug Administration's experts on soy, who stated that "there is abundant evidence that some of the isoflavones found in soy, including genistein and equol, a metabolize of daidzein, demonstrate toxicity in estrogen sensitive tissues and in the thyroid. This is true for a number of species, including humans."[51]

⊙ **Soy is filled with phytoestrogens.** Phytoestrogens are substances that can interact with your endocrine system and may cause a whole host of hormonal complications.[52]

⊙ **Soy is not good for infants, either.** A study published in the *New Zealand Medical Journal* estimated that the phytoestrogens in one day's worth of soy infant formula are the equivalent (on a body-weight basis) of five birth control pills.[53] In lab studies, it was found that exposure to phytoestrogens before or directly after birth, including genistein (which is present in soy), caused adverse reproductive issues later in life, including altered ovarian development, altered estrous cycles, problems with ovulation and infertility.[54]

⊙ **Soy is one of the foods most heavily contaminated with pesticides.** When you eat plants sprayed with pesticides, you inevitably ingest the pesticides, too. Pesticides are neurotoxins designed to kill living creatures. There are many cited negative effects of pesticides on humans, which may include damage to the nervous system, reproductive system and particular organs; immune-system dysfunction; a disruption of hormone function; and developmental and behavioral abnormalities. The more you avoid pesticide-sprayed crops, the better off you will be.

Fermented organic soy products, like miso, tempeh and natto, are acceptable to eat. The long process of fermentation (similar to how fermentation allows beneficial bacteria to flourish in raw sauerkraut) deactivates the trypsin inhibitors in soy in a way that cooking cannot and makes these products more easily digestible. Nama shoyu is a "raw," unpasteurized soy sauce made of fermented soybeans. However, nama shoyu contains gluten. I prefer and now exclusively use low-sodium tamari, which is also fermented but has the added bonus of being gluten- and wheat-free. Small amounts of tamari, along with occasional tempeh and miso consumption are the only soy products in my diet. Edamame, which are green immature soybeans, contain fewer of the toxins mentioned in these studies, so they can be enjoyed occasionally if you really love them.

All this means you'll want to avoid tofu, soy milk, commercial energy bars, soy burgers, soy cheese and other processed products containing soy protein isolates, soy protein concentrate, texturized vegetable protein or hydrolyzed vegetable protein. You will be much better off without these products. If you are unsure of a product, check the ingredients list.

EAT BEAUTY FATS IN MODERATION

There are many different types of fats:

- **Saturated fats:** Found in meat and dairy products, as well as some plant sources, like coconut oil.

- **Unsaturated fats:** Often referred to as "heart-healthy fats," these are found in plant sources, like avocados, nuts, seeds and olive oils, as well as in fish.

- **Trans-fatty acids or trans fats:** Unsaturated fats that have been altered through the process of hydrogenation. Considered the worst kind of fat, trans fats have been associated with heart disease and other health issues. These types of fats are extremely harmful to your health and beauty and should be avoided in all quantities.

Fat has some important functions, such as helping to make your skin supple and beautiful, lubricating your joints, protecting your cell membranes from oxidative damage, and helping to protect and insulate your nervous system. You also need some fat to absorb fat-soluble nutrients, including beautifying vitamins A, D, E and K. But you'll be getting enough fat, in the form of avocados, seeds and nuts, so that you don't have to seek it out. Avoid overdoing even "healthy" fats, though. I'll eat half an avocado or an ounce of nuts, but I don't eat them both at the same time. Cultures that eat low-fat diets, such as rural China, where the average dietary fat intake is 15 percent of calories, stay much thinner than Americans,[55] who average around 34 percent of calories from fat.[56]

Oil is extremely dense and contains no fiber, as the aforementioned fat-containing whole plant foods do. Getting the fat your body needs in limited amounts from whole plant foods, which contain fiber and come in a complete nutritional package, is far better than consuming oils. Oils are isolated from the food source they are derived from, and are therefore processed and not found naturally in nature. All oils should be strictly limited in your diet. In recent years, the media has popularized the consumption of certain plant oils, like flaxseed oil, as a good source of healthy unsaturated fat. But oil is still oil, no matter how you slice it—or, in this case, pour it. Virtually all my salad dressings in Part III are oil-free, and the other recipes that use small amounts of oil are spread over several portion sizes.

One more thing before we discuss some beauty fats in detail: fatty acids are the main building blocks of fats. Just as there are nine essential amino acids, there are two essential fatty acids that must come from foods: omega-3 and omega-6 fatty acids. Most people get too much omega-6 fatty acid, which is present in foods like vegetable oils and margarine, but not enough omega-3. You will get omega-3 fatty acids from consuming one to two tablespoons a day of chia seeds, hemp seeds or ground flaxseeds, which will further ensure you get your daily dose of omega-3 essential fatty acids. You need these for proper brain and nerve functioning.

Omega-3 fatty acids are converted into longer-chain EPA and DHA fats, which are considered "nonessential," since they can be made from the omega-3 fats found in greens, seeds and nuts. However, people's ability to convert the omega-3 fatty acids into DHA may vary. Taking an algae-based DHA supplement is good nutritional insurance, the way that a high-quality multivitamin also is. I do not recommend taking fish oil pills, which are often rancid and contaminated with toxins. Algae is the primary source from which the fish obtain their DHA.

AVOCADOS

Technically a fruit, avocados are a wonderful source of fat for your Beauty Detox. Dr. Norman Walker calls avocados "just about the finest fat we can put in our bodies."[57] With their creamy texture and beautifying oils, avocados are extremely filling and provide long-burning fuel. For a quick lunch, I'll layer some avocado slices on a few nori wrappers (the black seaweed that sushi is wrapped in, which you can get at health markets) with sprouts and lots of baby spinach, squeeze some lemon on them and wrap them up. A super-easy, filling and healthy lunch made in about one minute.

If you're used to eating a heavier diet, you'll find avocados a savior and a good replacement for meat and dairy products. For optimal health and especially when you're trying to lose weight, you must limit all fat, so half of an avocado a day is the maximum amount you should consume.

NUTS AND SEEDS

We've already discussed raw nuts and nut butters in detail in the protein section, but they also contain healthy beauty fat. Nut and seed pâtés are great staples for heavier meals. Nuts and seeds should always be soaked first and rinsed to remove inhibitor enzymes, which make them more difficult to digest. Because nuts are already dense and rich in protein and fat, it is best to enjoy them as the heaviest food in a meal and not combine them with avocados or concentrated animal protein of any kind. Check out some of the recipes in Part III.

Free Radicals and Antioxidants

Free radicals are atoms or groups of atoms that have at least one unpaired electron and become unstable and highly reactive. They are created as a result of the process of oxidation; that is, when a substance combines with oxygen due to a wide variety of internal and environmental stresses, such as exposure to pollution, chemicals and radiation. Free radicals are believed to cause tissue damage at the cellular level—harming your DNA and cell membranes, and accelerating the aging process.

Antioxidants are substances that may protect cells from the damage caused by free radicals by working to stabilize them. Examples of antioxidants include beta-carotene, lycopene and vitamins A, C and E, all of which can be found in plant foods.

COCONUT OIL

As I discussed, oil should be a very, very small proportion of your diet. But if there is a dessert or dish where you need a small amount of oil, coconut oil is a great choice because it has a higher smoke point than other oils and has some beneficial properties. In other words, because it's nearly a completely saturated fat, it's much less susceptible to heat-induced damage and will stay stable at higher temperatures. Coconut oil in small amounts is what I bake with instead of butter, vegetable oil or vegan butter, which contain vegetable oils (see the "Cut Back on Polyunsaturated Fats" section in this chapter).

Coconut oil is a unique oil. About 50–55 percent of the fatty acids in coconut oil are lauric acid, which can help support and restore your thyroid. In their book, *Virgin Coconut Oil,* Brian and Marianita Shilhavy point out that although coconut oil is a saturated fat, it is cholesterol-free and trans-fatty acid–free and has actually been shown to help lower cholesterol levels due to its ability to stimulate thyroid function.[58] Virgin coconut oil is composed of medium-chain fatty acids, or triglycerides (MCTs), which are shown to have many health benefits, including raising the body's metabolism, and acting as an antiviral, antifungal and antibacterial agent. Virgin coconut oil is the best natural source of MCTs, besides human breast milk. For more info on coconuts and coconut oil, see Part II.

Besides unrefined coconut oil, some oils that are okay to consume occasionally in their unrefined state are flaxseed, olive, pumpkin seed, hemp seed, borage seed and evening primrose. Honestly, though, I never use any of these oils except for olive, which is useful in tiny amounts for some recipes. It is vital that you consume these oils in a totally unrefined state. If they've been refined in any way, which could include processes such as bleaching or deodorizing, these oils are much harder on your liver to process. Unrefined oils don't contain preservatives. It is best to purchase them in dark glass bottles and keep them capped immediately after use, as light and oxygen can cause oxidation. They may be pricier than commercial oils, but your liver and your skin deserve the best, so consider this an investment in yourself and how you look and feel!

CUT BACK ON POLYUNSATURATED FATS

The fat-free craze of the 1980s, which instilled fear that any amount of fat makes you . . . well, fat . . . is as misguided as the more recent Atkins/super-high-animal-protein revolution. You need a small amount of fat in your diet to become your most beautiful and healthy. But it's crucial for you to weed through all the misinformation and distinguish between the types of fats that truly allow your cells to perform at their optimum potential, and the types of fats that destroy your beauty.

Most people know that margarine, hydrogenated oils and trans-fatty acids of all kinds, as well as refined oils, are some of the worst kinds of fat to consume. In addition, saturated fats and dietary cholesterol from animal products should be eliminated or strictly limited, because excessive dietary cholesterol can weaken the liver and is associated with health issues like heart disease and high blood cholesterol levels.

But because polyunsaturated vegetable oils have the word *vegetable* in their name, you might mistakenly think they are good for you. They are not. They, too, are among the most aging and beauty-squashing foods, and you want to eliminate them from your diet. That is why I never consume vegan butter spreads or vegan mayonnaise products, which are usually composed of virtually all vegetable oils.

Examples of oils containing polyunsaturated fats include:

Canola oil 32%	Safflower oil 77%*
Corn oil 62%	Soybean oil 61%
Cottonseed oil 52%	Sunflower oil 69%*
Grapeseed oil 70%	

*High oleic safflower and sunflower oils are produced from hybrid plants and have smaller amounts of polyunsaturated fat and higher amounts of monounsaturated fats, and are therefore more stable. But it's difficult to find truly cold-pressed varieties of these oils that have been stored and transported in completely refrigerated, protected conditions.

Polyunsaturated vegetable oils are now included in processed foods that range from rice milk to crackers, granola, roasted nuts and frozen waffles. Many restaurants use them and fast food joints proudly boast that they fry their French fries in vegetable oil, as if that were a good thing. Over the past century, vegetable oil consumption—namely, soy, corn, safflower and canola oil—has increased significantly.

The excessive consumption of polyunsaturated oils has been linked to many health issues and diseases, including damage to the liver, increased cancer and heart disease, immune-system dysfunction, damage to reproductive organs and lungs, digestive disorders, depressed learning ability, impaired growth and weight gain.[59] Polyunsaturated vegetable oils are extremely unstable (they are missing more than one hydrogen bond), and this instability gives way to reactivity, meaning they become rancid and oxidize when exposed to heat, air and light, and also simply as time passes and they sit in your cupboard. Rancid and oxidized oils are aging bombs that you don't want to ingest into your body, if staying young and beautiful is one of your goals. When you consume rancid or oxidized oils, they spew out the very thing you and I are trying to avoid: free radicals. Free radicals are like wearing a beautiful dress and having a torrential downpour completely drench you—hair, makeup, outfit and all. They destroy your beauty, causing DNA/RNA damage, as well as destruction to pretty much all the tissues in your body, from cell membranes to the collagen on your face. They wrinkle your skin and cause you to age prematurely.

Even when you first pick up that bottle of commercial vegetable oil from a neatly stacked pile at the supermarket, you may be buying oil that's already rancid to some degree.

It may already have been sitting in a warehouse for months, transported on hot trucks and waiting on the shelf for weeks unrefrigerated often in clear bottles that allow for light exposure, all of which provide lots of opportunity for it to oxidize. These oils may not look or smell rancid, but that's because they may be bleached and deodorized with even more heat to cover up any rancid smell. What's more, some polyunsaturated oils are low-yield, so solvents like hexane can be used to suck more oil out of them. As you can imagine, some of this toxic solvent can be left in the product that you then ingest.

Cooking with vegetable oils is where it gets really ugly. I literally cry when I see food demos on TV where they cook with what they generically refer to as "vegetable oil," teaching thousands of unknowing viewers to do the same. The heat forces the polyunsaturated molecules to react with oxygen and generate one free radical after another, creating a free radical cascade. Imagine a waterfall, but one spewing beauty-squashing molecules that inflict damage such as inflammation, a disruption of normal metabolic function . . . and yes, premature aging. It's like cooking with a liquid labeled "aging potion."

You may be wondering whether unrefined, hexane-free, cold-pressed polyunsaturated varieties of grapeseed oil or canola oil are okay. Chances are, you've heard that grapeseed oil is good to cook with because it has a high smoke point, or that canola oil is a healthy oil. Grapeseed oil (which I used to use) does have a fairly high smoke point. But at 70 percent polyunsaturated fat for grapeseed and 32 percent for canola, these are still highly reactive polyunsaturated oils that can react and create free radicals not only from heat, but from light, air and storage. So you can't just rely on an oil's smoke point to decide whether it's a good oil choice. Now I avoid them all and just cook with vegetable broth or coconut oil, or olive oil at lower temperatures. I also use a tiny amount of sesame oil for flavoring rather than cooking.

But even in the case where you might use high-quality, unrefined grapeseed oil and refrigerate it right away, you should still think twice about using it regularly. Why? Grapeseed and other vegetable oils are high in the omega-6 essential fatty acid (linoleic acid), which is already in overabundance in the average diet. You already get enough of it without even trying because it's prevalent in most foods, even in processed ones. Too many omega-6 fats can throw off your omega-6:omega-3 essential fatty acid ratio. Artemis Simopolous, M.D., who directs the Center for Genetics, Nutrition and Health in Washington, D.C., and is widely regarded as an expert in fatty acids, states that, "The ideal ratio is one to one or two to one, omega-6 to omega-3. Unfortunately, the American diet has been flooded with omega-6 fatty acids, mostly in the form of vegetable oils."[60]

Recently, researchers from the National Institutes of Health published an analysis of studies going back more than forty years. The research found that omega-3 fats linked to most of the heart disease protection, while a diet high in omega-6s may actually increase cardiovascular risk.[61]

The bottom line? Polyunsaturated oils are not beautifying. Avoid them, except for a tiny amount of sesame oil, which can be added to dishes for flavor but should not be used for cooking. Whole foods like sunflower seeds are great, but not their oil. There's no need for the neutral-flavored other ones in your life, especially when you have much better oil choices, like coconut and olive oil, available to you.

GET YOUR BEAUTY MINERALS AND ENZYMES

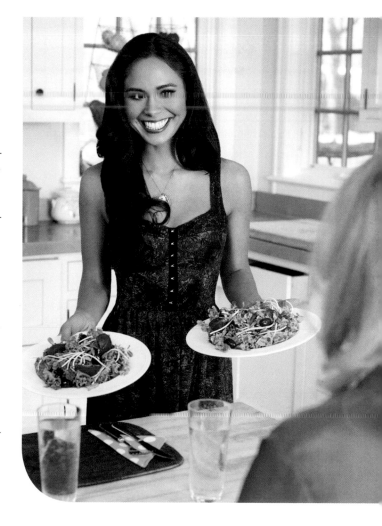

Minerals are one of the keys to beauty, and an incredible 95 percent of your body's activities involve minerals. Likewise, enzymes are the catalysts for hundreds of different processes in the body, including the rebuilding and renewal of skin collagen. Certain enzymes don't become truly active until the right quantities of trace and major minerals are present. And you need living, active enzymes to fully absorb and assimilate your beauty minerals. Minerals and enzymes are best friends.

ESSENTIAL BEAUTY MINERALS

Where do minerals come from? They primarily come from the soil, which is why the quality of soil is so important, and why you want to buy as much organic produce as possible, since organic soil has a higher mineral content than traditional farming soil. Some studies show that there are up to 87 percent more minerals in certain organic fruits and vegetables.[62] The minerals filter into plants through the water in the soil, which contains a wide spectrum of soluble minerals that are absorbed into plants, then move through the plants' stems and out into their leaves. Eating plants is like eating pure mineral content. (The only way you could get a more direct source of minerals is if you ate the dirt. But don't worry, we don't have to do that. You can get what you need from a much more appetizing source—fresh, juicy, green vegetables.)

Green plants are the number-one food group for providing you with all the minerals you need for superior beauty and nutrition, while simultaneously giving you the vitamins and the amino acids that you need to build protein. If you eat greens abundantly and get a good variety of them in your diet, you will inherently get the wide spectrum of minerals you need into your body. Greens are also among your strongest Beauty Detox weapons, because their powerful alkalinity helps root out poison the more consistently you consume them.

ENZYMES BUILD BEAUTY

In the mainstream health world, you often hear about measuring a food's worth by its protein, calorie and carbohydrate content. But what about enzymes? Dr. L.T. Troland of Harvard University said, "Life is something which has been built up about the enzyme; it's a corollary of enzyme activity."[63] And to that quote, I'd like to add that enzymes are also a major secret to beauty.

Live enzymes are the catalyst for every human function. As Dr. Edward Howell, one of the fathers of food-enzyme research, said, "the *length of life* is inversely proportional to the *rate* of exhaustion of the *enzyme potential* (that is, a supply of enzymes) of an organism."[64] Scientists have identified over 5,000 different enzymes that your body utilizes and manufactures, but there may be far more.[65] Enzymes are catalysts of biochemical reactions in living beings and perform thousands of important life-supporting functions. For example, enzymes help repair your DNA, help digest your food, and help you assimilate the nutrients within food. They repair and prevent wrinkles, help even out your skin tone, and contribute to smooth and youthful skin. Enzymes also help speed up weight loss and detoxification as they free up more metabolic energy. You need as many enzymes as possible to support these functions. You were born with a huge enzyme reserve, but this reserve decreases over time, causing aging and a slowing of the metabolism. Dr. Meyer and his research associates at Michael Reese Hospital in Chicago found that the enzyme level in adults aged twenty-one to thirty-one was thirty times greater than in adults aged sixty-nine to one hundred.[66]

The goal with Beauty Detox Foods is to preserve as many of your enzymes as possible. Think about it: if you have fewer enzymes working for you, their priority has to be the major processes that help you to stay alive, like digestion and blood rebuilding. Enzymes are essential for your vitality and increase your Beauty Energy. If you had a plentiful supply of enzymes in your system, the enzymes would be able to tend to both the major processes as well as repair those that affect the way you look, such as limp hair and crow's feet around the eyes. One way to do this is to infuse your body with enzymes, which are found in raw plant foods. The more of this living fuel you eat, the more alive you'll feel.

Enzymes are heat-sensitive entities. Although they hold up pretty well in the freezer, they become denatured and damaged at about 118 degrees Fahrenheit, and die at temperatures just above that. Take a look at a bunch of vibrant green kale. It's so incredibly thick and waxy that when you go to wash it, the water molecules slide right off. Now sauté that kale, and watch how the very vibrancy of the leaves fades. The leaves acquire a soft consistency and absorb water. Their enzymes have broken down.

This is not to suggest that you must eat 100 percent raw foods. Easily digestible cooked food has its place, too, and will still provide minerals and other nutrients. But it does mean that you should increase the percentage of raw greens and vegetables you consume overall. It is important to consume raw plant foods at the beginning of every meal (see Chapter 2). That could mean some Glowing Green Smoothie, a salad or a few celery sticks. Starting each meal with these raw greens and other veggies will ensure that you're increasing your enzyme intake. This alone will start rebuilding your beauty.

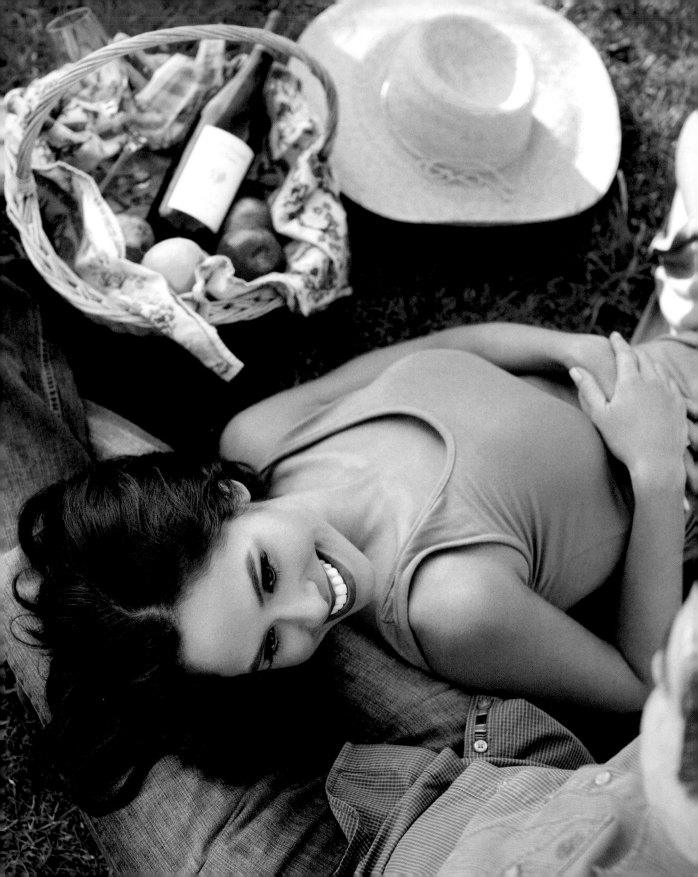

FINDING YOUR BEAUTY PHASE

3

In this chapter, you'll discover three phases of beauty: Blossoming Beauty, Radiant Beauty and True Beauty. Blossoming Beauty starts you on a new way of eating, while giving your body time to adjust. You may decide to start with Radiant Beauty, which builds on the Blossoming Beauty principles, adding the Glowing Green Smoothie and reducing your intake of animal products. This is the phase in which you'll see incredible results in your skin, under-eye circles and hair. In the True Beauty Phase, which some people decide never to visit, you may drink Glowing Green Juice as well as the Glowing Green Smoothie, and may decide to eliminate all animal products from your diet. But if it's the right phase for you, you'll be rewarded with a very high level of health and beauty.

TRANSITIONING

Transitioning your diet is critically important. Consider that you've probably spent at least a few decades eating acidic foods, the residue of which is lodged as sludge, in varying degrees, in different parts of your body. If you decide to make a radical shift to a diet with a high percentage of alkaline foods—namely, fruits and vegetables—you are also unleashing the strongest possible cleansers that you can put into your body. Beauty Detox Foods are going to wake up sleeping demons in the form of toxic waste. You want to wake up a limited amount of toxins at a time, which can then leave the body in a controlled way. If you don't do this, you might experience very unpleasant side effects, such as headaches, nausea, dizziness, breakouts and other skin eruptions, and diarrhea, and actually feel quite sick. You may even feel bloated or heavier, because your body is holding on to more fluids to help neutralize acids. This is why it's essential to transition your diet properly. It is absolutely critical to incorporate the cleansing methods discussed in Chapter 2. I cannot stress that strongly enough. Eliminating waste is as important as changing your diet.

Beauty Detox Foods are not something you adopt for twenty-one days or a few months, only to go back to your old ways. This is a lifestyle, a long-term way of eating, so it's crucial to understand how important it is to pace yourself throughout this process. It's easy to get really enthusiastic and want to do a complete overhaul of your diet immediately. That's what happened to me. I was so fascinated with the concepts I was learning that I made drastic changes overnight. I didn't suffer any severe trauma, but I did hit physical and mental roadblocks and detox walls along the way, which I want to help you avoid.

If toxins don't leave the body quickly, or at all, what you've done is reawakened poison and brought it to the surface, where it will be reabsorbed by the tissues. The three phases—Blossoming Beauty, Radiant Beauty and True Beauty—take this into account. Transitioning your detox from phase to phase is critical, as are the cleansing methods. But no matter what phase you are in, you will see results.

Stick to It!

You are improving as long as you don't give up. Focus on progress, and don't think you have to be perfect. Stick to the phase you're in, and if you stray, get right back on the path. Keep your bigger goals in mind. Visualize how you want to look and feel and hold onto that clear picture. This information has come into your life for a reason. Use your inner strength and power, which you already have within you, to harness this knowledge to improve your health and start glowing from the inside out. Start nourishing your body properly today, and claim the health and beauty you deserve.

Consider these guidelines for transitioning:

◉ **Stay in each phase at least one month before moving on.** If you're feeling good in a certain phase, you can stay there for as long as you want. You will improve at any level, although you may see the most radical change when you progress to (or begin at) Radiant Beauty and start enjoying the Glowing Green Smoothie. When you want to achieve better results, you can move forward to the next phase. The degree to which you want to improve, and the current state of your health, will dictate how quickly you move up to a different phase.

If you are losing weight and feeling good, but that requires debilitating discipline—you are constantly dreaming about and obsessing over food—you are not ready to move up yet. Drop down to the next level or stay where you are for as long as it feels comfortable and natural. Stay in a phase until you don't have to think about it anymore, until it has become ingrained in your life. If you move up before then, you will feel deprived and you'll "cheat."

◉ **If you aren't seeing the results you want, focus additional efforts on cleansing.** Along with eating well, cleansing your body is critically important to clear out toxins and waste, so that you can absorb more beauty nutrients from the healthy foods you're eating. Be sure you're incorporating probiotics and digestive enzymes, magnesium-oxygen supplements and/or other cleansing methods I mentioned in Chapter 2, and lots of Probiotic & Enzyme Salad. You'll also want to get gravity colonics or do at-home enemas. Remember that cleaning your body of sludge is just as important as what you put into your body.

⊙ **Avoid feeling judgmental and competitive with yourself, or attacking yourself for feeling weak at times.** Remember that you are creating a whole new lifestyle that is meant to last the rest of your life. Take your time transitioning. Be kind to yourself.

⊙ **Keep things simple.** What you need more than anything is salads and lots of greens. You have to retrain yourself to regard salad as the main part of your meal, not as an appetizer or a side dish.

You may feel overwhelmed if you believe you have to throw out everything in your pantry and fridge and go shopping for all new items. You don't have to. Instead of getting overwhelmed with recipes, focus on creating a few basic salads and other recipes in Part III that you love and that can be your staples.

⊙ **View desserts as occasional treats.** I've included some dessert recipes to enjoy in moderation. They are all sweetened with natural ingredients, like stevia and raw coconut nectar, and are gluten-free and vegan, so they all digest pretty cleanly. But that is not to say they should be eaten daily or often—they should not be.

What about Supplements?

Supplements should *never* be deemed a substitute for a healthy diet packed with fresh greens and other produce. You do not need to and should not buy a million different pills. However, I recommend taking a high-quality, whole-food-based and nonsynthetic multivitamin supplement as good insurance. It should include vitamin D_3 (which most people need to supplement) and the spectrum of B vitamins, including vitamin B_{12}. And if you're vegan, you should definitely supplement vitamin B_{12}. Other than that, be sure to pick up a probiotic supplement, digestive enzymes, a magnesium-oxygen supplement and chia, hemp or flaxseeds for daily omega-3 fats. An algae-based DHA supplement is also further good insurance, as some people don't convert omega-3 fats adequately into longer-chain DHA fats.

BLOSSOMING BEAUTY
ONE-WEEK MENU SUGGESTIONS

In this phase, not only do you not have to buy any new kitchen equipment, but many of the foods are upgraded variations of foods with which you are already familiar. Using more favorable ingredient substitutions, as well as incorporating abundantly more green vegetables, means you will still make significant progress. You will have more energy and less bloat, and you will lose weight, especially in the belly area.

Animal products can be kept in your diet, except for dairy, but should be consumed only once a day at a maximum. You'll cut out highly refined sugars and carbs, and start to wean yourself off gluten-containing foods, like wheat, rye and barley, which can cause bloating and are difficult to digest. By starting to cut out gluten you will automatically cut out junk food, since so much processed food contains wheat and wheat derivatives. But you won't miss any of those foods, anyway, as you'll be eating beauty grains, such as quinoa and millet, and products made of them, such as bread, crackers and pasta. For now, we're limiting all sugars, which includes fruit. The only fruit allowed in Blossoming Beauty are low-sugar fruits: lemons, limes, cucumbers, tomatoes. Grapefruit and some green apples (like Granny Smith apples) are okay, too.

If you are more than fifty pounds overweight, are exhausted, suspect you have candidiasis, have a lot of skin issues and/or are an absolute beginner, I recommend starting with Blossoming Beauty. If these concepts seem totally foreign to you and you're used to eating various forms of animal protein every day, Blossoming Beauty may be the right place to start. If you don't have any of the issues just mentioned, you might just try diving into Radiant Beauty.

The dishes mentioned in this menu are suggestions. You do not have to make all of these recipes, but follow the general guidelines of what and how to eat at each meal. Additional recipes can be found in Part III. Dishes that are italicized can be found in Part III.

FIRST THING IN THE MORNING

Cup of hot water with the juice of half a lemon

1 probiotic supplement with a pint of water

BREAKFAST

16–24 ounces *Glowing Green Smoothie, Low Sugar*, or

2–3 celery stalks

If you are still hungry or choose not to have the smoothie,

YOUR CHOICE OF

- *Raw Rolled Oat Cereal*
- *Buckwheat Gluten-Free Vegan Pancakes*
- *Gluten-Free, Low Sugar Sprouted Buckwheat Granola*

- 1–2 pieces of toasted, plain, gluten-free bread (with 1 Tbs. of avocado as a spread, if necessary)

- Cooked oatmeal, topped with cinnamon and sweetened with stevia, as needed
- *Energy in a Spoon*

LUNCH

A digestive enzyme

Large green salad, such as *Earthy Oregano Kale Salad*, with one of the dressings in Part III

YOUR CHOICE OF

- *Healthy French Onion Soup* with gluten-free crackers or 1 piece of toasted gluten-free bread

- *Portobello Mushroom Burger*
- *Creamy Cashew-Free Veggie Korma*
- *Spicy Baked Sweet Potato French Fries*

- *Southwestern Savory Root Vegetable Latkes*
- *Smoky Eggplant, Herb and Cabbage Soup* over *Simple Spiced Quinoa*

SNACK

- Veggie sticks with your choice of salsa or *Raw Muhammara Dip*
- *Power Protein Smoothie*
- *Glowing Green Smoothie, Low Sugar*
- *Energy in a Spoon*
- *Fresh PR Coconut Meat Yogurt*

DINNER

A digestive enzyme

Large green salad with one of the dressings in Part III

$1/2$ cup *Probiotic & Enzyme Salad, Ginger-Caraway Variety* or *Kimberly's Kimchi*

YOUR CHOICE OF

- *Green Spring Vegetable Risotto*
- Lightly steamed broccoli and baked fish (see page 16 for a list of fish considered lower in toxins) with lemon
- Baked or roasted chicken; lightly sautéed spinach (in vegetable broth) with garlic
- *Black Bean Burritos with Spicy Red Sauce*
- *Gluten-Free All-Veggie Pizza*
- Quinoa pasta with *Homemade Bella Marinara*
- *Spanish Millet Paella*
- Veggie omelet made with two organic eggs
- *Sesame Seed–Tempeh Gorilla Wraps*
- *Baked Spicy Sweet Potato French Fries* and *Rosemary Cauliflower "Mashed Potatoes"*

LATE NIGHT

Herbal tea with stevia (optional)

Veggie sticks with salsa (only if you absolutely need something to chew)

1 probiotic supplement with a pint of water

2–4 capsules of magnesium-oxygen supplement (follow directions and, if diarrhea develops, reduce amount). Can be used on an intermittent basis.

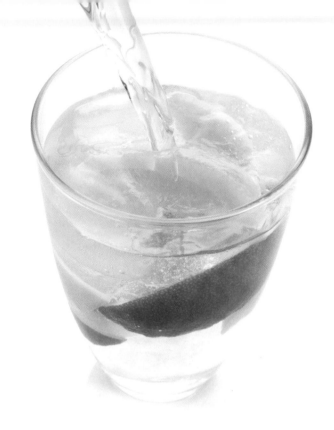

RADIANT BEAUTY
ONE-WEEK MENU SUGGESTIONS

In this phase, you start enjoying the classic Glowing Green Smoothie, which is super-exciting! Your mornings will extend the "cleanse mode" that your body has been in through the whole night, so that the hours that you are cleansing start to add up on a daily and weekly basis, and you are consistently getting more sludge out of your system.

You'll reduce your intake of animal products further, but you can still have them a few times a week, especially fish lower in toxins (see page 16) and eggs. You will have some beautifying fats from avocados, seeds and nuts, as well as beauty grains and the products that come from them.

This is the phase where you may experience the biggest results and lose the most weight. Your skin will glow and become smooth, your under-eye circles will diminish, and your hair will shine.

FIRST THING IN THE MORNING

Cup of hot water with the juice of half a lemon

1 probiotic supplement with a pint of water

BREAKFAST

16–32 ounces *Glowing Green Smoothie*

If you're still hungry after 30 minutes, occasionally on mornings that you are really active, woke early, or are simply starving, try one of these:

- ¼ cup *Gluten-Free, Low-Sugar Sprouted Buckwheat Granola* with or without unsweetened almond milk

- *Raw Rolled Oat Cereal*
- Cooked oatmeal, topped with cinnamon and sweetened with stevia, as needed

- *Energy in a Spoon*

LUNCH

A digestive enzyme

Large green salad, such as *Earthy Oregano Kale Salad* or *Raw Brussels Sprout Salad*, with one of the dressings in Part III

YOUR CHOICE OF

- *Asparagus and Leek Soup*
- *Tom Kah Thai Coconut Soup*
- *Raw Corazon Chili*

- *Simple Spiced Quinoa* and steamed broccoli to top your salad
- *Yin-Yang Meal: Baked Squash, Steamed Kale and Quinoa Pilaf*

- *Raw Zucchini Pesto Pasta*
- *Cracked Caraway Seed, Brussels Sprout, Squash and Carrot Stew over Brown Rice*

SNACK

YOUR CHOICE OF

- *Power Protein Smoothie*
- More *Glowing Green Smoothie*

- *Endurance Protein Bar*
- Veggie sticks with salsa or *Raw Muhammara Dip*

- *Energy in a Spoon*
- *Fresh PR Coconut Meat Yogurt*

DINNER

A digestive enzyme

Large green salad with one of the dressings in Part III

½ cup *Probiotic & Enzyme Salad, Ginger-Caraway Variety* or *Kimberly's Kimchi*

YOUR CHOICE OF

- *Cumin Chili Chickpea Burgers*
- *Quinoa Ten-Veggie "Fried Rice"*
- *Asparagus and Veggie Tempeh Stir-Fry over Kelp Noodles*
- *Italian Eggplant Caponata* and baked fish (see page 16 for a list of fish considered lower in toxins) with lemon

- *Shiva-Shakti Daal* over brown rice
- *Spinach-Basil Polenta with Creamy Sauce*
- Veggie omelet made with two organic eggs
- *Raw Asian Creamy Kelp Noodles*
- *Stuffed Acorn Squash*

- *Probiotic-Boosting Polish Borscht* with a side of *Simple Spiced Quinoa*
- *Smoky Tempeh over Sautéed Broccoli Rabe*
- *Sweet Potato Shepherd's Pie*

LATE NIGHT

Herbal tea with stevia (optional)

1 probiotic supplement with a pint of water

2–4 capsules of magnesium-oxygen supplement (follow directions and, if diarrhea develops, reduce amount). Can be used on an intermittent basis.

TRUE BEAUTY
ONE-WEEK MENU SUGGESTIONS

In this phase, you'll drink Glowing Green Juice as well as the fiber-containing Glowing Green Smoothie, or just stick with the GGS, if you like. You'll reduce the amount of animal products in you diet to only a small portion of fish, eggs and goat's cheese, eliminating land animals altogether. Once you get to this point, you may decide that you don't want to eat any animal products at all.

You'll eliminate cooked grains not only in the mornings but generally also at lunch and in the middle of the day, which keeps your inner tract even more clear and accelerates cleansing for longer periods.

This is a pretty advanced level of diet that may not work for everyone's lifestyle or genetic makeup. If you moved to this phase from Radiant Beauty but simply find it to be a daily struggle and too much effort, or feel too deprived or too obsessive about your diet, move back down to the Radiant Beauty Phase, which might be the right phase for you over the long term. But if the True Beauty Phase feels right to you, you'll be rewarded with a very high level of health and beauty.

FIRST THING IN THE MORNING

Cup of hot water with the juice of half a lemon

1 probiotic supplement with a pint of water

BREAKFAST

16–30 ounces *Glowing Green Juice* or *Glowing Green Smoothie*

If you're still hungry after 30 minutes, follow with a piece of fresh fruit or the *Glowing Green Smoothie* (or more of it)

Energy in a Spoon

LUNCH

Large green salad with one of the dressings in Part III

YOUR CHOICE OF

- *Jicama, Cucumber, Papaya and Lime Salad* topped with ½ an avocado
- *Spiralized Asian Veggie Salad*
- *Smoky Eggplant, Herb and Cabbage Soup*

- *Rosemary Cauliflower "Mashed Potatoes"* (cooked or raw version)
- *Raw Purple Cabbage Slaw* with *Raw Brussels Sprout Salad*
- *Roasted Portobello*

- *Mushroom and Creamy Dijon-Arugula Salad*
- *Raw Herb Tastes-Like-Real Stuffing*
- *Blueberry and Avocado Salad*

SNACK

YOUR CHOICE OF

- 8–20 ounces *Glowing Green Smoothie* or *Glowing Green Juice*
- ¼ cup *Gluten-Free, Low-Sugar Sprouted Buckwheat Granola*

- Veggie sticks with salsa or *Raw Muhammara Dip*
- Fresh fruit (be sure there's been at least 3–4 hours since you've had any nuts or seeds)

- *Power Protein Smoothie*
- *Energy in a Spoon*
- *Fresh PR Coconut Meat Yogurt*

DINNER

A digestive enzyme

Large green salad with one of the dressings in Part III

$^{1}/_{2}$ cup *Probiotic & Enzyme Salad, Ginger-Caraway Variety* or *Kimberly's Kimchi*

YOUR CHOICE OF

- *Quinoa, Squash, Avocado and Microgreen Timbale Stacks*
- *Jenna's Baked Falafel* topped with *Creamy Dijon-Tahini Dressing*
- Lightly steamed broccoli and baked fish (see page 16 for a list of fish considered lower in toxins) with lemon

- *Gluten-Free Vegan Lasagna Supreme*
- *Raw No-Bean Refried Beans*
- *All-Green and Tempeh Calcium Stir-Fry*
- Veggie omelet made with two organic eggs
- *Kale, Carrot, Pinto Bean and Quinoa Stew*

- *Lentil-Mushroom Tarts*
- *Yin-Yang Meal: Baked Squash, Steamed Kale and Quinoa Pilaf*
- *Raw Gorilla Taco Wraps*
- *Black Bean Burritos with Spicy Red Sauce*

LATE NIGHT

1 probiotic supplement with a pint of water

2–4 capsules of magnesium-oxygen supplement (follow directions and, if diarrhea develops, reduce amount). Can be used on an intermittent basis.

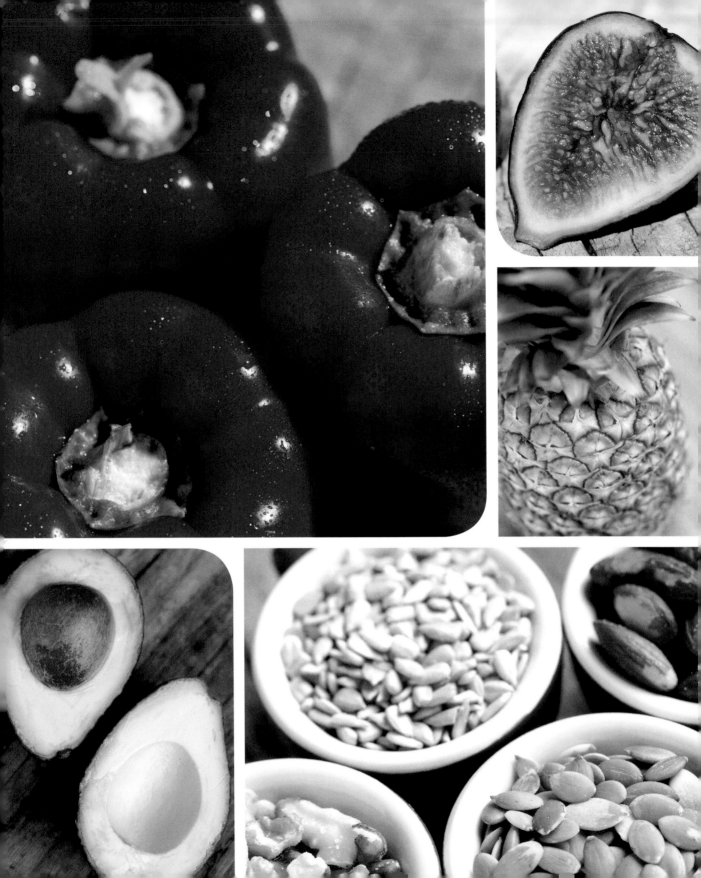

BEAUTIFUL SKIN

4

Across every culture in the world, and from the days of Cleopatra to modern times, one beauty trend remains the same: the desire for smooth, beautiful skin. Beautiful skin is so sought after that many women spend more resources on beautifying this feature than all other aspects of beauty combined. But after spending copious amounts of money on products, they ignore the powerful impact their diet has on their skin. Now *you* can take control and transform your skin. Combine excellent skin care with powerful beauty foods, and watch how beautiful your skin will become.

Check out the online Resources section at www.kimberlysnyder.net to see the brands and skin care products I recommend.

YOUTHFUL SKIN

It is obvious from the vast quantities of anti-aging creams, facial procedures and injections on the market that smooth, supple skin is the holy grail of beauty. Although you may be spending a lot of money on skin products, you may not be feeding your skin properly from the inside. The best way to rejuvenate your skin depends on the right combination of key nutrients (see Part I).

It's possible that many of the foods you've been eating a great deal of to lose weight or keep a toned body, show up right on your face in the form of wrinkles. Foods that age the body—namely, excessive amounts of meat and dairy products—age the skin. In Part I, I mention Dr. Hiromi Shinya, the chief of the surgical endoscopy unit at Beth Israel Medical Center, and clinical professor of surgery at Albert Einstein College of Medicine, both in New York City. After examining the stomachs and intestines of hundreds of thousands of patients, he wrote in *The Enzyme Factor,* "Once you reach a certain age, your body's growth changes into a phenomenon called aging. Eating meat may accelerate growth, but it will also speed up the aging process."[1]

Dr. Shinya points out that a diet including excessive animal protein creates toxic by-products that can damage the DNA, put an excessive burden on the liver and kidneys, create calcium deficiencies and osteoporosis, and result in a large loss of energy. That's why people who eat high-protein diets may get hard bodies, but they also get hard, lined faces.

Would you want to be a size two but look ten years older than you are? If you want to keep your skin as young-looking as possible, you must reduce your meat intake to a maximum of ten to fifteen percent of your overall diet (or eliminate it altogether), eliminate dairy and increase your consumption of plant foods, while simultaneously cleansing your body of mucus and toxins. That's the real secret to youthful skin.

Age Spots

The skin is a window reflecting the inside of the body. When you see liver spots or brown aging spots on the skin, their size and prevalence may not only be indicative of sun damage from overexposure, as commonly believed, but also an indication of how much damage free radicals from oxidation have done to the inside of your body. This brown age pigment, called lipofuscin, is a mixture of free radical–damaged fats, proteins, sugars and metals.[2] It is a waste by-product of worn-out cells that are not eliminated from the body. Besides avoiding overexposure to the sun, you can help prevent more oxidation from occurring and perhaps even reduce the spots you already have by consuming the right foods and avoiding fried foods, animal fats, polyunsaturated vegetable oils and refined sugars.

BEAUTY FOOD 1: RED BELL PEPPERS

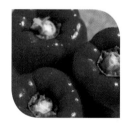

Red bell peppers are fantastically high in vitamin C, which helps repair and regenerate collagen, the protein that gives structure to your skin. Technically a fruit, these brilliantly colored peppers are low in sugar and higher in nutrients than other types of peppers. Red bell peppers are a good source of the mineral silicon, which diminishes wrinkles and makes skin more supple and youthful. If you're deficient in silicon, it shows up as sagging skin that's neither resilient nor strong. The connective tissues throughout the body are made up of collagen and elastin, which are strengthened by silicon. Eating red bell peppers helps to keep them healthy and supple.

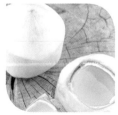

BEAUTY FOOD 2: COCONUT

Coconut in all its forms, including its water, meat, and oil, is one of the finest beauty foods available to promote youthfulness. Coconut is technically a drupe, which is a fruit with a hard stony covering enclosing the seed.

Whenever I go to tropical places around the world, including the Pacific islands, the Caribbean, Southeast Asia and Mozambique, I consume coconuts daily. There's nothing I find more delicious than drinking the water from a fresh coconut, seconds after it is chopped from a tree and opened in front of me. Coconuts have been used in Ayurvedic medicine and Hindu rituals, and in the Philippines, the coconut is commonly called the "tree of life."

You can eat and drink from young coconuts found in your health or Asian markets, as I often do. If this isn't convenient for you, boxed coconut water is now commonly found in markets everywhere. It is still one of the best natural hydrators there is, especially if you're active. Your skin must be hydrated to look younger, which will also aid in the healing and rejuvenation of skin's collagen, and help restore elasticity and flexibility to your skin. Dehydration can make the skin look dried out, withered and leathery, and may lead to dark under-eye circles, collagen damage, wrinkling and other signs of premature aging.

The key nutrients contained in coconut water include lauric acid, iron, potassium, magnesium and calcium. Potassium, an electrolyte that facilitates cellular cleansing, is about twice as concentrated in coconut water as in a banana. The soft, young coconut meat is moisturizing and nutrient-rich, and certain cultures believe it has healing, youth-promoting qualities.

The oils you consume and cook with may be one of the biggest culprits in accelerating aging in your diet. As I discuss in Chapter 2, polyunsaturated vegetable oils are unstable and can oxidize quickly, creating free radicals that make you age faster. By contrast, coconut oil does the opposite. However, it should still be used sparingly, as with all other oils. Coconut oil is a unique type of saturated fat made of medium-chain fatty acids that are digested differently than other types of oils. They're broken down and converted into energy in the body, rather than tending to be stored as body fat.

Because coconut oil is saturated, meaning it doesn't have any missing hydrogen atoms that can break easily to form free radicals when heated, coconut oil stays stable at high cooking temperatures. When I do cook with small amounts of oil—albeit infrequently—I use coconut oil almost exclusively, including for occasional baked and raw dessert treats. It can help normalize blood sugar levels, reduce adrenal work (and therefore exhaustion, which helps reduce under-eye circles), increase Beauty Energy and reduce the amount of digestive work that is required by your system.

Coconut oil disrupts the lipid membranes of viruses, bacteria, yeast and fungi and helps destroy them. Therefore, it is also very useful to those with candidiasis, acne or other skin conditions, like psoriasis, that may be aggravated by these viruses, bacteria, yeast and fungi.

A few decades ago, a lot of misinformation was promulgated that coconut oil is harmful to heart health. But the truth is that the people of the Pacific Islands whose traditional diets are high in coconuts have very little cardiovascular disease.[3] In fact, studies have shown that coconut oil doesn't adversely affect cholesterol levels and destroys both the bacteria and viruses most associated with atherosclerosis, which can lead to plaque formation and heart issues.[4]

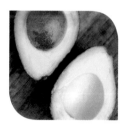

BEAUTY FOOD 3: AVOCADOS

Sometimes the look and consistency of a particular food hints at its amazing beauty benefits. Avocados are one such food. Their yellow interior is luscious and creamy. If you eat avocados often, you will see your skin start to soften and become more supple and youthful. I've been eating avocados regularly for years now as an essential part of my regimen to keep my skin looking its best. If I'm working in a desert environment, such as in southern California or New Mexico, I increase my consumption of avocados.

Avocados have long been noted among cultures in Central and South America, such as the ancient Maya Indians, for their powerful anti-aging effect on the skin and joints. Avocado's abundant monounsaturated fats are ideal for skin rejuvenation and moisturizing from the inside out, preventing premature wrinkling. Avocado oil is close in composition to our natural skin oil. Its fats are also useful in lubricating the digestive tract, promoting the absorption of fat-soluble vitamins in your tissues and making your cellular membranes stronger.

Avocados are full of compounds that nourish skin health and help maintain youthful skin tone. They're also rich in the skin-smoothing beauty vitamins: A, C, E (the best source of any fruit) and K. Look to avocados for minerals such as potassium, copper and iron, the last two being mineral constituents of antioxidant enzymes. They also contain an amino acid known as glutamine, which helps to protect your skin from environmental damage, and glutathione, an antioxidant that researchers have found to be important in preventing aging.[5]

Avocados have one of the highest amino acid contents of all fruit, building protein in the body. Although avocados have a relatively high fat and calorie content, it's a gross oversimplification to say "fat is fat" and not evaluate how cleanly (or not) a particular fat is digested, in terms of deposits it leaves behind in body. The raw plant fat in an avocado is digested very efficiently (as opposed to rancid polyunsaturated fat, for instance) and is extremely nutrient-dense per calorie. Still, around half of an avocado or one small one is the maximum amount that should be consumed daily.

At around ten grams of fiber, avocados contain large amounts of both soluble and insoluble fiber, which has the youthful and slimming ability to assist with ongoing cleansing. In studies, avocados have been shown to have a favorable impact on cholesterol.[6] The combination of good fat and fiber helps control blood sugar levels. These qualities, along with a high concentration of minerals and vitamins, make avocado a food that can help prevent you from binging on foods high in refined sugar or that contain rancid fats, which are the real foods that make you gain weight and that destroy your skin.

Oxalic Acid

Some research shows that oxalic acid, which is in a variety of foods such as caffeine products, cola drinks, asparagus and certain greens, including spinach, can bind in some plants and prevent some calcium absorption. However, the degree to which this occurs is controversial. In the book *Human Nutrition and Dietetics*, Stanley Davidson points out that the chelating effect of oxalic acid on minerals like calcium is most likely negligible.[7] Gabriel Cousens, M.D., author of *Conscious Eating,* postulates that upon examining the oxalate sediment in hundreds of people's urine, the oxalate from natural foods do not build up in the system if digestion and fat metabolism are working properly.[8] In *Fresh Vegetable and Fruit Juices,* Dr. Norman Walker says that when greens are cooked (rather than eaten raw), oxalic acid binds irreversibly with calcium, hindering its absorption and crystallizing in the kidneys.[9] This is a controversial, unresolved issue, so the best idea is to rotate your raw greens, including spinach, to ensure that all foods in your diet are balanced.

BEAUTY FOOD 4: SPINACH

Spinach is an all-around skin beauty power food. It's rich in beta-carotene, which converts to the powerful anti-aging vitamin A. This important nutrient promotes youthful skin by allowing for proper moisture retention in the epidermis, helping to prevent wrinkles, removing dead skin cells from your body and making room for fresh new ones. Spinach also contains lipoic acid, which helps antioxidant vitamins C and E regenerate—those important nutrients needed to maintain youthful skin.

Spinach has concentrated health-promoting phytonutrients, such as carotenoids and flavonoids, to provide you with powerful antioxidant protection against damaging free radicals. It also contains vitamin K (one cup contains more than your daily requirement), as well as numerous beauty minerals, including manganese, calcium, magnesium, zinc, folate and selenium. Its rich content of these nutrients, plus plentiful amino acids and about twice the fiber in other greens, makes it a top beauty choice to add to your Glowing Green Smoothies and salads.

Non-heme iron, which is the plant-based form of iron, is a component of blood hemo-globin, which carries oxygen to all body cells. Healthy blood and blood flow are necessary for youthful, glowing skin. Non-heme iron is best absorbed in the presence of vitamin C, and thankfully, spinach contains both these nutrients.

Enjoy spinach both raw and cooked. In its raw form, such as in the Glowing Green Smoothie, you will enjoy its full range of the important beauty vitamins, especially vitamin C, which is destoyed by heat.

Recipes for Youthful Skin

RADIANT SKIN

I can't help it. I notice the skin of everyone I meet: waiters, drugstore checkout employees, people on the subway and those sitting next to me in the park, in yoga class or in line at the market. Unfortunately, dull skin is far more common than radiant skin. Dull skin has the inevitable effect of undermining your beauty. It is impossible to truly hide dull skin behind mineral-infused foundation and shimmery highlighters.

If you currently have dull skin, you can create a beautifully radiant complexion with the Beauty Detox lifestyle changes. The foods in this chapter, along with the entire Beauty Detox program outlined in Part I, will help eradicate dull skin and replace it with lustrous, velvety luminescent skin. And looking radiant can make you *feel* radiant, which can change your whole outlook on the world, and change the way the world looks at you.

BEAUTY FOOD 5: WATERCRESS

Watercress is a spicy member of the mustard family, and it helps create glowing skin. Its pungent taste is combined with the ability to cleanse and oxygenate tissues. When your body has an increased oxygen supply, you have better blood flow and more glowing skin. Watercress has an array of minerals, including calcium and iodine, that help remineralize your body and prevent deficiencies that equate to a dull complexion. Also high in vitamins A, C and E, watercress is useful in treating skin issues, such as acne and eczema.

A highly alkaline green vegetable, watercress helps neutralize acidic waste products throughout the blood and lymphatic system. It contains mustard glycosides, which can invigorate circulation and enhance healthy blood flow to help cleanse more toxins from the body.

When I was recently working on a film in New Mexico, I found watercress growing abundantly next to the natural springs where I was hiking. Picking it from the clear, fast-moving springs by the handful and eating it fresh was an incredibly satisfying experience.

BEAUTY FOOD 6: FIGS

The tiny seeds of figs are packed with nutrients that help cleanse the digestive tract of toxins and mucus. Figs are one of nature's best laxatives. In *The Mucusless Diet Healing System*, Professor Arnold Ehret includes charts from physiological chemistry food researcher Ragnar Berg of Germany, which pinpoint figs as a top

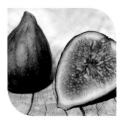

mucus-dissolving food.[10] Dissolving mucus, toxins and waste from the body and blood are vital to enhancing the inner glow that shows up in your face. Additionally, excess mucus in the digestive tract may be preventing vital nutrients from getting to the skin.

You can eat them plain, or add them to your Glowing Green Smoothie when they're in season. A Vitamix blender is strong enough to pulverize the seeds, helping to release the stored antioxidants and polyphenolic bioflavonoids stored within them. This is the way to get the most nutrition and beauty benefit out of figs.

Fresh figs are in season from July through September, which is when I buy them and eat them regularly. I also occasionally enjoy dried figs, which can be used in moderation as a natural sweetener for desserts and smoothies.

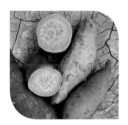

BEAUTY FOOD 7: SWEET POTATOES

If your skin is looking dull and lackluster, especially in the middle of winter, eat some brightly colored foods, which will impart some of their radiance to you. Sweet potato is an excellent starchy vegetable to include in your diet, as it contains the magical skin-brightening combination of vitamin A and vitamin C. Together, these antioxidant vitamins work to neutralize cell tissue–damaging free radicals.

The sweet potato's brilliant orange color is attributed to its high levels of carotenoids and beta-carotene, which the body converts into vitamin A. Sweet potatoes can also help protect against cancer, heart disease, and inflammation-related health issues, such as asthma and arthritis. Sweet potatoes are also rich in biotin (vitamin B_7) and vitamins B_2, B_6 and E. They are a healthy source of iron, potassium (which helps keep the right fluid balance in your body's cells), copper, manganese and folate.

Sweet potatoes are easily digested, and because they're relatively low in sugar, compared with other starchy root vegetables, and high in fiber, they help to maintain stable blood sugar. They pair well with other veggies and salads. Try my Ganesha's Sweet Potatoes and Italian-Style Sweet Potatoes recipes in *The Beauty Detox Solution*, as well as Creamy Cashew Free Veggie Korma and Sweet Potato Shepherd's Pie in Part III.

Choose sweet potatoes that have the deepest orange color, which indicates the highest carotene content. Be sure to eat organic ones with the skin on, as the skin contains a good amount of fiber and nutrients.

BEAUTY FOOD 8: CUCUMBERS

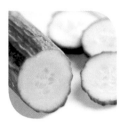

Cucumbers are high in enzyme-charged water, B vitamins, nutrients and electrolytes to build skin radiance from within. Other key beauty minerals cucumbers contain are potassium, calcium, iron, and magnesium.

The silica found in abundance in cucumber skin is necessary for reaching your maximum potential for a glowing complexion, and makes your skin resilient and radiant. The naturally filtered, enzyme-rich water in cucumbers makes them an excellent hydrator, which is needed for supple skin.

Besides water, the flesh of cucumbers is made up of vitamin C, which further contributes to bright skin, and caffeic acid, which has anti-inflammatory properties and is soothing to the skin. This is why cucumber slices have been commonly used to help reduce under-eye puffiness, and why you may have them placed over your eyes in a spa treatment.

Cucumbers can help prevent sad, dull skin on other parts of your body as well. Try rubbing a few slices of cucumber directly onto problem cellulite areas for a few moments. The phytochemicals in the cucumber cause the collagen in your outer skin layer to tighten up, reducing the visibility of cellulite, so don't forget to pack some for your next pool party. Cucumbers even help flush out the kidneys and prevent bloating all around the body.

I always emphasize starting meals with some type of raw food, such as a green salad or some veggie sticks, because these contain an abundance of enzymes, water and fiber that help you fill up on the good stuff, promoting ideal digestion and keeping you from overindulging in skin-dulling foods, such as dairy and heavy, refined starches. Cucumber is one of the best of these foods, since it has such a high water content, plus fiber. Be sure to buy organic cucumbers, which are free of pesticides and the waxes that make peeling non-organic cucumbers necessary. Organic cucumbers can and should be enjoyed with their full skin intact, which allows you to get the full dose of beautifying silica.

BEAUTY FOOD 9: ACAI

Acai is one of the few foods on the beauty food list that's grown in only one part of the world: South America. Although I like to include foods that can be widely sourced, acai is included because it's so commonly found today in health markets, and its skin-boosting benefits are truly worth taking note of.

Acai is the top antioxidant-rich fruit, with research showing that acai has 500 percent more antioxidants than blueberries. This makes it a power food for brightening dull skin. Acai's superior antioxidant content comes from anthocyanins, which are responsible for acai's brilliant purple color, and flavonoids, along with antioxidant vitamins. Dull skin looks even worse if it appears withered and malnourished. Acai's power nutrients have a renewing effect on the complexion, while also protecting against aging and skin-damaging free radicals.

Although acai is a berry, it's actually a fatty fruit, containing omega fatty acids that help to nourish skin cells. These fatty acids also work to help ensure that fat-soluble beauty vitamins are being absorbed into the body and are getting to the skin. It has a high amount of vitamin C to brighten skin, and vitamin E, which helps smooth the skin to help it look more radiant. Acai also contains minerals, such as potassium and calcium. As if that weren't enough to pack into these little power berries, acai also contains energizing B vitamins and has a good amount of fiber, which helps keep your system free of the toxins that can cause clogging and prevent nutrients from getting to your skin.

You can find acai packets in the freezer section of your local health store, where they have been flash-pasteurized and frozen soon after being picked, so they're as close as possible to being raw and still contain most of their nutrients. Try the Power Protein Smoothie in Part III.

Recipes for Radiant Skin

SOFT SKIN

Dry skin cries out for nourishment and hydration from within. The stratum corneum is a thin outer layer of skin composed of dead cells that are held together by lipids, which are fatty compounds. If this thin outer layer is weakened, the cells take longer to be replaced, from the lower range of four weeks up to six or eight weeks.

The easy thing to do is slather on heavy creams but, ironically, many of such creams are drying to the skin (see "The Ideal Skin Moisturizer" sidebar). Many skin care products, especially thick, heavy face creams, rely on inexpensive oils and synthetics to make the skin feel moisturized. But they may just sit on the skin's surface, limiting respiration, hindering natural regeneration processes and promoting free radical buildup—all major causes of skin aging. Cheap petroleum-based ingredients, like mineral oil, for example, can be likened to trans-fatty oils in foods: they hinder the skin from breathing to its maximum extent and expelling toxins.

Choosing the right skin care products is important. But so is eating properly, and moisturizing your skin from within is critical to achieving the soft, supple skin you're after.

The Ideal Skin Moisturizer

Commercial creams contain a great deal of water. All this water is readily absorbed into dry skin, expanding the tissues and making you think your skin is becoming more moisturized. But as soon as the water evaporates, the dry skin comes back.

Be especially aware of lotions and products that contain polyunsaturated oils—there are a lot of those products out there. Just as they can age you by ingesting them (see Chapter 2), they can age you when you put them on the surface of your skin, where they can oxidize and form free radicals, especially if the product also contains petroleum-based ingredients, which keep the product sitting on the surface of the skin longer. Be sure if a product contains such oils the manufacturer is using the highest quality, and is processing and storing them at cold temperatures. Cheap filler and petroleum-based ingredients can also be toxic and aging.

By contrast, using natural products, such as coconut oil, as a body moisturizer makes your skin more youthful by providing deep and real moisture. It helps strengthen underlying tissues and helps remove excessive dead cells on the skin's surface that makes your skin rough and flaky in texture.

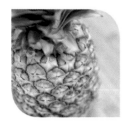

BEAUTY FOOD 10: PINEAPPLE

Pineapple is excellent in promoting efficient digestion, which is what soft, beautiful skin is dependent on. Pineapple possesses high levels of a special protcolytic enzyme called bromelain. Proteolytic means "breaks down protein." Bromelain promotes the breaking down of protein and foods throughout your system, and cleans the blood by removing debris and toxins from the bloodstream.[11] Poorly digested toxins and by-products of digestion that continue to recirculate around the body can lead to wrinkles and hardening of the face. Because of these properties, ripe pineapple further helps to reduce gas and excessive gastric acids in the body,[12] making it helpful as an anti-bloating food.

Pineapple's bromelain enzyme is also believed to be helpful in improving circulation and reducing mucus,[13] which are key components to ongoing cleansing and detoxification, which keeps skin soft and healthy. Bromelain is also considered an effective anti-inflammatory. Inflamed skin and tissues do not look soft or youthful. It also helps discourage blood clot development. In Germany, bromelain is approved as a post-injury medication because it is believed to reduce inflammation and swelling.[14]

Pineapple is also high in vitamin C, which helps in the formation of collagen, a protein that helps grow new skin and blood vessels. Natural vitamin C in fruit can help mitigate the effects of sugar and fructose in the body that pineapple and other fruits also naturally contain.[15] Pineapple contains manganese, which is a critical mineral in keeping skin healthy and promoting skin healing, which also helps regulate blood sugar levels. Only one cup of freshly cut pineapple will supply you with nearly 75 percent of the recommended amount of this mineral.[16]

I love pineapple and eat ample amounts of it very often, either in the late morning if I get up early and want a snack before lunch, or in the middle of the afternoon.

BEAUTY FOOD 11: ALMONDS

Almonds are a wonderful aid for dry skin, and may even be useful for other skin issues, such as psoriasis. Almonds are an extremely rich source of the skin-beautifying antioxidant vitamin E, the major antioxidant in human epidermal tissue, which creates smoothness and suppleness. Research indicates that vitamin E may help fight the signs of aging by helping protect your skin against the damage caused by ultraviolet rays, while nourishing the skin from elements that can cause dryness.[17]

Almond oil is a renowned skin moisturizer, and by consuming almonds, you'll help nourish your dry skin from the inside out. Almonds contain monounsaturated fats that help soften and protect the skin. These fats are an important part of your cell membrane, and they keep skin from losing its own natural moisture and drying out. Almonds also contain minerals, including zinc, calcium (more than any other nut), iron, potassium, manganese, magnesium, selenium, copper and folate. They're full of amino acids to build protein in the body. They also provide some of the B vitamins. An analysis conducted at Tufts University showed that a handful of almonds contains levels of flavonoid antioxidants on par with broccoli and green tea.[18] All pretty impressive for a little nut!

In traditional Chinese medicine, almonds are used as a tonic, are considered anti-inflammatory, and are known as brain and bone food, probably thanks to their high content of calcium and other key nutrients. They're believed to prevent stagnation of *chi* in the liver. In Ayurvedic medicine, almonds are used to strengthen *ojas*, which is the Sanskrit word for vigor, and are said to promote self-control, give life energy and soothe the nervous system.

Pairing almonds with the right foods can increase their benefits even more. Research shows that vitamin E and vitamin C work better together to make your skin more beautiful. I recommend pairing almonds with plant foods high in vitamin C, such as in or after a salad of dark leafy greens with lemon. Also try the Power Protein Smoothie, which combines almond milk with acai, a fruit that's high in vitamin C (acai is a fatty fruit that digests well with proteins), Raw Herb Tastes-Like-Real-Stuffing and Raw Corazon Chili, all in Part III.

BEAUTY FOOD 12: WALNUTS

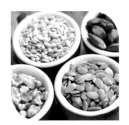

If you rub a shelled walnut between your fingers, you will feel its natural oils on the surface of your skin. Walnuts boast the highest content of omega-3 fatty acids (an important beauty fat) of any nut. Omega-3 fats keep the cellular membranes flexible and fluid, optimizing the cell's ability to usher in nutrients and moisturizing fluids to prevent dryness and to help eliminate wastes. As you saw in Part I, you want *more* omega-3 fatty acids and fewer omega-6 fatty acids in your diet, so that your body's systems function at their peak (see Chapter 2).

Walnuts are rich in vitamin E, which helps protect dry skin from the harsh elements of the environment, and are high in protein, fiber, some B vitamins, magnesium, calcium and potassium. They're also a very good source of both manganese and copper, two minerals that are essential cofactors in a number of enzymes that are important in antioxidant defense. The powerful oxidative enzyme superoxide dismutase, which neutralizes damaging free radicals produced within the cells, requires manganese and copper. Walnuts also contain L-arginine, an amino acid that helps with the healing and repair of collagen and tissue.

Finally, you know that beauty sleep contributes to radiant, supple skin. Walnuts naturally contain melatonin, a hormone that helps ensure good sleep and helps increase antioxidant activity.

I don't use walnut oil because I always recommend eating the whole walnut to get the benefit of its fiber content. Check out my Raw Gorilla Tacos in Part III—the perfect, delicious way to get more walnuts into your diet.

BEAUTY FOOD 13: FLAXSEEDS

As you incorporate flaxseeds into your diet, you'll notice your skin becoming smoother, healthier and more nourished. Flaxseeds also contain vitamin B_6, calcium, magnesium, folate, iron, zinc and manganese, and some research has shown they have cancer-fighting properties.

Because flaxseeds contain among the highest level of fiber in any food (both soluble and insoluble forms), they are a real winner. Flaxseeds stabilize blood sugar, promoting cleansing. It is important to keep the body cleansed of wastes so that nourishing nutrients can reach the cells of your body, including your skin.

Flaxseeds offer vital omega-3 fatty acids that supply the right ratio of essential fatty acids to your body, ensuring peak functioning. Omega-3 fatty acids also help prevent inflammation, which can lead to dry and damaged skin.

I recommend eating flaxseeds in their whole form, which includes the fiber, rather than using flaxseed oil. For optimal freshness, soak flaxseeds overnight in water, rinse well and then grind them in a spice grinder right before consuming them. Flaxseeds are prone to oxidation if stored for too long or with exposure to excessive heat or light. They are best stored in the fridge.

Recipes for Soft Skin

UNLINED, WRINKLE-FREE SKIN

Considered inevitable by those who don't want to resort to fillers, surgery or Botox, deep lines can be softened considerably through the smoothing effect of certain foods. People who have deep lines often eat a great deal of congesting foods, such as meat, shellfish and dairy, which contain no fiber and move much more slowly through the digestive tract. As you clear blockages in the colon, the lines on your face may start to lighten. I've personally experienced this, and I've seen improvement in my clients. When I look at pictures of myself in my early twenties, when I ate a lot of clogging foods like skinny lattes, tofu, pretzels and mozzarella, my nasio-labial lines between my nose and mouth were much more pronounced than they are now (thankfully!). Sure, aging is a natural part of life, but we can eat our way to minimizing its visible signs.

BEAUTY FOOD 14: PEARS

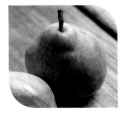

This easy-to-find fruit is supportive of both the lungs and the colon, so it's perfect in targeting the deep nasio-labial line via the Chinese face-mapping theory, which considers the lungs and colon yin-yang organs. This is also why pears are an ingredient in the Glowing

Green Smoothie. They're believed to improve lung function and even help reduce Chronic Obstructive Pulmonary Disease symptoms such as breathlessness and coughing, and they're said to be useful in treating inflammatory conditions of the mucous membranes. An Australian study has revealed the consumption of whole pears has a protective effect against developing asthma.[19] Most of the fiber in pears is insoluble, making them a colon-cleansing food. At 5.5 grams of fiber, a medium pear is a high-fiber food that helps cleanse the digestive tract of aging toxins and wastes before they show up on your face as lines.

In addition, pears possess the powerful beauty vitamins C and E, along with some B vitamins and vitamin K. They are also a good mineralizing fruit, containing copper, manganese, potassium, iron, magnesium, selenium, calcium, zinc and folate. Although pears have a high ORAC (oxygen radical absorbance capacity), which neutralizes aging free radicals quite efficiently, most of pears' antioxidants are contained in the skin. For this reason, be sure to purchase organic pears whenever possible, so that you can eat the skins.

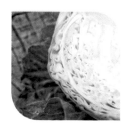

BEAUTY FOOD 15: CABBAGE

Humble and inexpensive, cabbage perfectly exemplifies that Beauty Foods don't always have to be exotic, rare or even particularly beautiful themselves (although when I cut one open, I find the countless layers in a cabbage sort of mesmerizing to look at). Cabbage contains the magical skin beauty triumvirate of vitamins A, C and E. It is not commonly known that cabbages actually contain about 11 percent more vitamin C than oranges by weight, and vitamin C is the super anti-aging nutrient that helps heal damaged tissues and minimize deep lines. Its vitamin A content is also useful in smoothing skin lines.

Cabbage is rich in sulfur, which is good for wound healing, and the combination of sulfur and vitamin C gives cabbage potent detoxifying qualities. It purifies the blood of toxins, such as free radicals and higher-than-normal levels of uric acid, which may contribute to the visible signs of aging, including deep lines. Sulforaphane, found in cabbage, augments the production of antioxidant and detoxification enzymes in the body.

Cabbage is high in fiber, so it clears the waste that congests in your internal organs (and then shows up on your face in the form of lines). Culturing your cabbage ferments its natural sugars (see the Probiotic & Enzyme Salad in Part III), which creates beneficial bacteria that help cleanse the digestive tract. While some lines are a natural form of aging, with a superior diet and ongoing cleansing to keep aging toxins from constantly circulating, you can help minimize, reduce and prevent many deep lines on your face.

Also a good source of iodine, cabbage is a good food for the thyroid and other endocrine glands. Cabbage is also helpful for proper muscle development and is rich in minerals, such as calcium, magnesium and potassium. The B vitamins in cabbage help soothe the nervous system and boost energy.

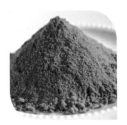

BEAUTY FOOD 16: TURMERIC

I first learned about turmeric in its place of origin: India. It is highly prized in Ayurvedic medicine for its health and beauty properties. It's a brilliant yellow that adds color to recipes and stains the skin, but I met Indian women who used to mix a little with sesame oil and apply it directly to their skin for beautifying benefits. Curcumin, which is the antioxidant flavonoid present in turmeric, has been gaining a lot of press lately in the Western world, as it has been shown to have anti-inflammatory effects, making it beneficial for the cardiovascular system, among other things.

Turmeric's beautifying properties are related to how it cleanses the blood. It keeps the red blood cells from clumping, promotes their formation, increases circulation and aids in tissue healing. Because it helps increase circulation via better blood flow, turmeric helps make the skin more glowing, supple and healthy-looking. Cleansed blood also helps prevent acne and skin disorders.

Recipes for Unlined, Wrinkle-Free Skin

CLEAR, BLEMISH-FREE SKIN

Zit. Pimple. Blemish. Breakout. Whitehead. Blackhead. If you have ever suffered from acne, as I have, you'll associate the experience with frustration, embarrassment and dread. Acne isn't simply just a superficial issue; it can destroy confidence, which is an important quality of magnetic beauty.

While I am a big advocate of using the right skin care products, many people use good products but still have chronic acne. You may be one of those people who has wondered why you can't get your pesky acne to vanish. The Beauty Detox approach to acne addresses the root cause, which concerns blockages within the internal organs, specifically in the liver and colon.

The liver filters toxins and usually pushes the waste into the colon. But when these organs become overloaded with waste and toxins, the toxins have to be pushed out through the skin, another eliminative organ, creating those ugly pimples. Acne is an external symptom of a much deeper issue. World-renowned endoscopic surgeon Dr. Hiromi Shinya, who has performed over 370,000 colonoscopies, points out, "No matter how good the food is, if you cannot excrete that food properly, it will rot and produce toxins in the intestine. Once it reaches this state, the balance of the intestinal bacterial flora will collapse in an instant. The reason you get pimples and rashes when you're constipated is that toxins, which get produced in the intestine, cannot be sufficiently excreted from the intestine."[20]

Perhaps it seems strange to you that your intestines, deep within your body, affect the skin on your face. But all parts of your body are interconnected. If you want to eradicate acne, you have to eliminate the root cause by minimizing toxicity in your body and maintaining ongoing cleansing of your digestive tract through better dietary choices. Cooked fats, especially polyunsaturated vegetable oils and dense animal oils, dairy products, and processed and refined foods that contain chemicals and preservatives are extremely difficult for the body to digest. They end up creating toxic substances that overwhelm the liver and colon. Certain medications, as well as hormonal changes, may also contribute to acne.

BEAUTY FOOD 17: PROBIOTIC & ENZYME SALAD

Probiotic & Enzyme Salad (see page 212) is extremely important in your ongoing efforts to eliminate acne naturally. There is no other food in my personal journey that has helped me maintain clear skin as much as this one. Probiotic & Enzyme Salad is loaded with probiotics, or good bacteria, and enzymes, as the name suggests. It is basically raw sauerkraut.

Probiotics have been associated with helping to keep the growth of unfavorable bacteria, yeast and fungi in check; keeping the immune system strong; ameliorating food allergies and inflammatory intestinal disorders; and helping to prevent constipation and other digestive problems.[21] Dr. Shinya calls "bacteria with antioxidant enzymes"[22] that neutralize free radicals within the depths of your body "good bacteria." When your intestinal flora is balanced and digestion is excellent, you get clear, beautiful skin.

I believe it's important to consume probiotics from a whole food–based source, and not just rely on supplements, though I do also recommend taking probiotic supplements. Probiotic & Enzyme Salad is a live, powerful beauty food that's made from the Beauty Food cabbage. You may also hear of good bacteria being associated with yogurt, but see Chapter 1 for the reasons that I don't recommend dairy yogurt. Probiotic & Enzyme Salad is also high in B vitamins, and helps your body manufacture and synthesize missing elements of the B complex family of vitamins right in your gut. Probiotics are important for synthesizing other essential nutrients as well, such as vitamin K, in the small intestine.[23]

Raw sauerkraut has been consumed for thousands of years. In fact, it's said that Chinese workers ate it while building the Great Wall of China and the Romans carried barrels of sauerkraut as protection against intestinal infections. I recommend eating at least half a cup daily at dinner. You can also buy raw sauerkraut in the refrigerated section of the health food store, but be careful of how much salt is contained in packaged brands.

BEAUTY FOOD 18: ARUGULA

Arugula is high in vitamin A, which not only protects the skin from free radical damage, but has been shown to be an anti-acne nutrient. Since a lack of vitamin A can lead to acne, it's important to load up on arugula, as well as other dark leafy greens that are high in vitamin A, such as watercress, broccoli and spinach.

A pungent, spicy member of the mustard family of dark leafy greens, arugula is highly alkaline, and helps cleanse and neutralize acidic waste throughout the blood and lymphatic system. Cleansing wastes from your body helps prevent toxic overload, a precursor to chronic acne outbreaks.

Arugula is also a good source of vitamins C and K, iron, calcium and fiber. I recommend pairing arugula in salad with avocado, so that the natural fats in the avocado balance arugula's peppery taste.

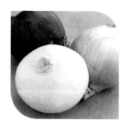

BEAUTY FOOD 19: ONIONS

Onions are beneficial cooked or raw, and possess antiseptic properties that cleanse the liver and skin. This humble but powerful Beauty Food contains flavonoids that stimulate the production of glutathione, which is the most important antioxidant the liver uses for detoxification.[24]

Onions have potent antibacterial properties, balancing bad bacteria in your body's inner ecosystem. They also contain a good deal of sulfuric oils, which stimulate the mucus lining of the sinuses and digestive tract.

Onions are a great blood cleanser, and they work by helping to thin the blood and eliminate clumps formed by fat, protein and sticky red blood cells. This allows more oxygen to flow efficiently in the bloodstream, which will help create a glowing, clear complexion.

Full of other beauty benefits, the humble onion is also high in usable quercetin, which is an antioxidant flavonoid that helps neutralize free radicals in the body, protects against heavy-metal damage, regenerates vitamin E and strengthens capillaries, which protects against varicose veins.

Some cultures believe that onions have potent longevity properties and consider them a type of natural medicine. Onions also contain vitamins A and C, sulfur, calcium, potassium, iron, silicon and fiber.

BEAUTY FOOD 20: RAW APPLE CIDER VINEGAR

Raw apple cider vinegar has long been honored for its many beauty and health benefits, one of which is as a natural antidote for acne.

I have noticed a definite link between constipation and acne in my clients. Raw apple cider vinegar is a strong digestive aid, helping to cure constipation and stimulating stomach acid, which aids in digestion. It also has antiviral, antibacterial and antifungal properties, which are of further benefit in dealing with candidiasis and yeast issues. Raw apple cider vinegar helps promote the growth of probiotics, the beneficial bacteria in your system, by acting as a prebiotic that feeds the probiotics in your digestive system.

This unique vinegar contains potassium and other trace minerals and elements. Because it helps balance the yeasts and bacteria in your body that feed off sugar, consuming it may help alleviate sugar cravings.

It has been theorized that raw apple cider vinegar is an effective weight loss aid, which speeds the metabolism and encourages fat-burning. It is even available in supplement form as a weight loss product.

Note how I keep using the word *raw,* which is what this type of vinegar must be in order for you to reap these benefits. Don't just buy any old apple cider vinegar you find at the supermarket or corner deli. Select one that's labeled "raw" and "unfiltered" or still contains the "mother," which implies that it's unpasteurized and has its own enzymes, beneficial bacteria and living nutrients. You'll find it at the health food store. It may cost a few dollars more than other vinegars, but thankfully it's not outrageously expensive.

I have found the benefits of raw apple cider vinegar are greatest when taken before meals. Two ways I suggest consuming it are first to include it in a Beauty Detox salad dressing or recipe (check out Part III of this book as well as *The Beauty Detox Solution*). I often use it in cooking to brighten dishes, instead of cooking wine. The other way is to dilute one tablespoon in a glass of water and drink it twenty minutes before your meal. Admittedly, I definitely prefer the first way!

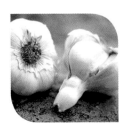

BEAUTY FOOD 21: GARLIC

Would you believe garlic can enhance beauty, not just repel people by creating bad breath, as commonly acknowledged? Well, it's true! Garlic purifies the bloodstream and enhances detoxification to help secure clear skin over the long haul. Garlic's effect on detoxifying the body and optimizing digestion is of particular importance. Garlic is a wonderful digestive aid, as it exerts a beneficial effect on the lymphatic system and aids in the elimination of noxious wastes from the body. It stimulates both secretion of digestive juices and peristalsis, the wavelike muscle contractions that move waste matter along through your digestive tract. Garlic also has an antiseptic effect and is an excellent remedy for infectious diseases and inflammations of the stomach and intestine.

The active component in garlic is the sulfur compound it contains, called allicin, a powerful natural agent that helps inhibit the ability of germs to grow and reproduce. In fact, it is said that one milligram of allicin has a potency of fifteen standard units of penicillin, which makes garlic a natural deterrent to internal yeast infections. Garlic can be useful for candidiasis, a condition that tends to accompany acne.

Garlic is an overall health-promoting food and research has shown it to help support the cardiovascular system.[25] It is packed with vitamins and nutrients, including potassium, B vitamins and vitamin C. Minerals such as potassium and many other compounds are believed to have anticancer properties.

BEAUTY FOOD 22: LEMON

If you want clear, glowing and blemish-free skin, make sure lemons are part of your daily diet. Lemon aids with digestion by increasing the secretion of bile from the liver, while also acting as a strengthening agent for the liver's enzymes. Any support to the liver, which is our primary detoxifying organ, is going to help clear up acne in the long run.

Lemon is high in vitamin C, which is water-soluble and travels easily through your body, destroying free radicals and toxins. Lemon acts as a blood purifier and as a cleansing agent to flush out bacteria and toxins in the body. These properties, which aid digestion, also make it helpful in long-term weight loss.

Although it has natural citric acids, lemon is actually alkaline-forming upon digestion (see Chapter 2 for more info on how foods digest to be either alkaline or acid-forming upon digestion). Lemon is a vitamin C–rich citrus fruit that helps bring a radiant glow to your complexion, fighting wrinkles and rejuvenating skin from within. It also contains the minerals calcium, potassium and magnesium.

An integral part of the Beauty Detox program is drinking hot water with lemon each morning—a potent way to increase lemon's benefits with a detoxification boost. I also recommend having lemon juice throughout the day, freshly squeezed in water and in salad dressings and recipes. Aim to consume the juice of two fresh lemons each day.

Recipes for Clear, Blemish-Free Skin

Glowing Green Smoothie	168
Glowing Green Juice	172
Ginger-Caraway Probiotic & Enzyme Salad	212
Roasted Portobello Mushroom and Creamy Dijon-Argula Salad	207
Baked Stuffed Veggie Eggplant	256
Oil-Free Garlic, Raw Apple Cider Vinegar, Tahini and Almond Butter Dressing	186
Quinoa Ten-Veggie "Fried Rice"	273
Homemade Bella Marinara	185

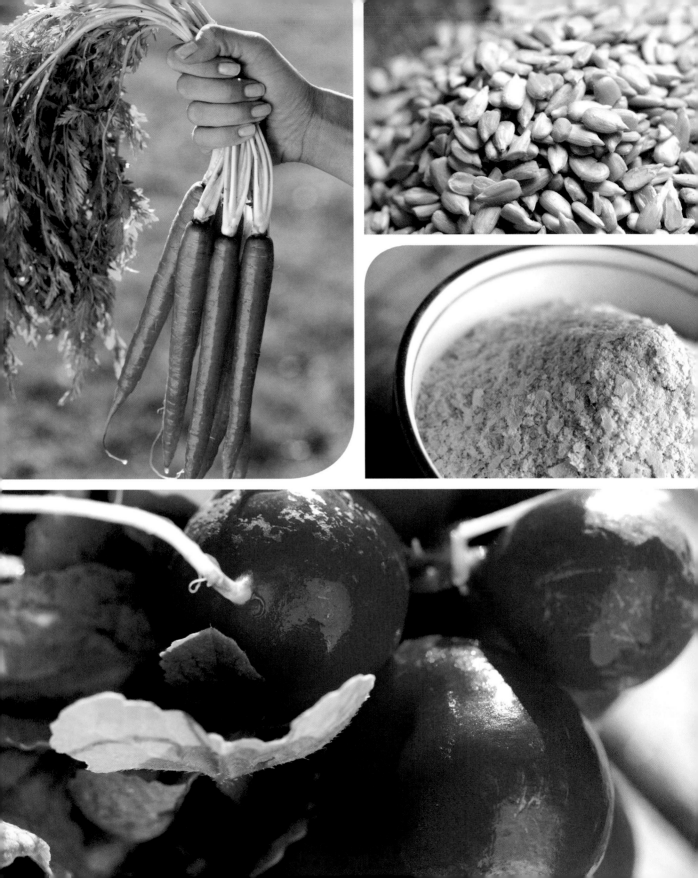

BEAUTIFUL HAIR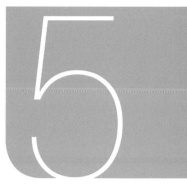

People always comment on how thick and healthy my hair is, but what they don't realize is that they're seeing the end result of a dramatic Beauty Detox transformation. Through my early twenties, my hair was a coarse, frizzy debacle of tresses that I had to constantly pull back into a bun. It was such a bummer! My diet of soy cappuccinos, pretzels, mozzarella and tomato paninis, and fake meat–filled Asian dishes were clogging my body and failing miserably at providing my hair the nourishment it needed to flourish.

When I overhauled my diet, my hair completely changed. It became softer and developed so much natural body that, to my absolute glee, it would bounce over my shoulders and down my back when I walked, instead of just hanging there like a heavy, lifeless curtain. It does take more time to see hair changes than it does to see changes in your skin, because you have to rebuild your hair follicle and hair grows only one-quarter to one-half inch per month. Give it a few months, and you'll find that eating the Beauty Detox way will change the body and health of your hair from within in a way that no salon treatment or product ever could. Your hair's healthy growth depends on the nutrients you put into your body, and the overall health of your body. When there are limited nutrients to go around, your hair will inevitably suffer, because your hair isn't an organ the body deems necessary for survival (of course, you may deem it necessary to have sexy, good hair for your social survival and simply for walking around in the world!).

Amino acids supplied from the right foods are also important, as hair is almost 97 percent protein. Gray hair can be caused by a lack of B vitamins, trace minerals such as silicon and sulfur and/or a deficiency of raw fatty acids. Beauty minerals such as sulfur, copper and silicon are also important to help keep the texture of your hair healthy and maintain its natural color.

Yet even if you ingest all these nutrients, they will never reach your hair if there is congestion in the body. Foods that don't digest cleanly—dairy, soy, wheat, polyunsaturated oils, animal fat and sugar—congest the body and can create toxins. If your blood becomes clogged with waste, the fine capillaries nourishing the hair follicle can get clogged. The entire blood and lymphatic system needs to be purified, cleansed and nourished in order for hair follicles to get the nutrients they need. That's why it's important for you to adhere to my ongoing cleansing regimen, recommended in Chapter 2, to help you grow that great hair.

Staying hydrated is also of utmost important, because water hydrates the hair strands from the inside out, nourishing new hair growth. And because your body will take care of your vital organs and tissues first, with limited water intake, your hair can get dehydrated far sooner than the rest of your body. Water also helps flush toxins from the body that can hinder your hair from growing in healthily.

Your hair sheds from the roots, and can break anywhere along the hair strand. Being dehydrated can cause more shedding and breakage, and also makes it harder for you to grow thicker, healthier and longer hair. Dehydration can also lead to scalp issues like dandruff, and can slow hair growth because there isn't enough moisture in the hair root to allow for healthy new hair growth.

Looking at Your Nails

Your nails indicate how mineralized your body is. Weak or ridged nails indicate mineral deficiencies. In ancient Eastern philosophy, some cultures believe that a lack of a white half moon in each nail bed indicates low circulation and vitality in the body. Be sure to eat Beauty Foods high in silica, which include millet and leafy green vegetables, as well as a wide range of plant foods high in minerals and vitamins to grow strong, healthy nails.

BEAUTY FOOD 23: PUMPKIN SEEDS

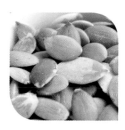

Take your cue from Native Americans in the 1800s, who ate pumpkin seeds as part of their traditional diet and had shiny, jet-black hair strong as a rope. Include pumpkin seeds in your diet to help ensure that your hair grows in robust and healthy—pumpkin seeds are one of nature's top hair-building foods.

Pumpkin seeds are an excellent source of zinc, sulfur (which is a mineral part of amino acids that protein synthesis depends on, as well as having detoxifying properties) and vitamin A. These three compounds, taken together, are particularly helpful in building strong hair. Because of their high zinc content, pumpkin seeds also help ward off acne and other skin imbalances. They contain B vitamins, which include biotin, an essential nutrient for strengthening hair, helping to prevent thin and brittle hair, and increasing hair growth.

Pumpkin seeds are a rich source of essential fatty acids, which nourish the scalp. (A dry, dull scalp can lead to dry, dull hair.) Last but not least, pumpkin seeds are also rich in cell-protecting vitamins C, E and K. Along with vitamin A, which you can get from other Beauty Foods like carrots (also discussed in this chapter), vitamin C is needed by your body to produce sebum, an oily substance secreted by your hair follicles that's your body's natural hair conditioner.

Pumpkin seeds supply a good amount of protein, along with magnesium, calcium, phosphorous, manganese, copper and iron, which build healthy blood flow to ensure optimal nutrient distribution to the hair follicle. Throw them into your salads or snack on them instead of peanuts or pretzels.

BEAUTY FOOD 24: DULSE

When I was first introduced to dulse (which rhymes with "pulse") by one of my nutrition teachers, I wrinkled my nose suspiciously and reluctantly tasted an amount the size of a rice grain. But now dulse is one of my favorite daily staples, and I find it absolutely delicious in its whole leaf form. Land vegetables are becoming more depleted in minerals as the soil quality diminishes, so sea vegetables supply an alternative way to reap the wide variety of beneficial minerals from the sea.

Dulse is an ancient health food that has been used by the peoples of Japan, Asia, Canada, Ireland and other Northern European countries for centuries. Adding dulse to salads is like adding a pure hair mineralizer—think of it as an ingestible hair product. Dulse will nourish your body and hair follicle with vitamins B_6, B_{12}, E and A, and is rich in iron, which promotes healthy blood flow to ensure that the nutrients get to the hair follicle. Other beauty minerals it supplies are zinc, calcium, potassium and magnesium, as well as iodine, which is a nutrient that is important for thyroid health.

Low in sodium but still possessing a naturally salty taste, dulse is a fantastic replacement for salt in salads and other recipes, in either whole leaf or flaked form. Dulse is a perfect travel food, as it comes dried and packs well. I've been known to add dulse to dull room-service salads and foods during press tours. It really perks up boring food and adds a huge hair beauty punch of nutrition.

You can find dulse in health markets, where it's increasingly common. Look for organic brands, which are tested for heavy metals to prevent contamination. I now greatly prefer the whole dulse leaves to dulse flakes; the flakes sometimes have a slightly fishy taste to some people. Dulse leaves ship well, so you can find them online if your local health food store doesn't carry them.

BEAUTY FOOD 25: CARROTS

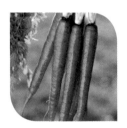

Carrots are well known as an important food for eye health, but you may not know that they should be part of your arsenal of top Beauty Foods to help create the gorgeous hair you're after.

Carrots have the highest amount of beta-carotene, the precursor for vitamin A, among the common vegetables. Vitamin A is necessary for a shiny, well-moisturized head of hair, as well as promoting a healthy scalp, which is essential for healthy hair growth.

Natural healers have long believed carrots possess strong cleansing properties that are effective in detoxifying the liver, helping to remove toxins from the blood to facilitate better transport of nutrients to nourish hair. Carrots also contain calcium, potassium, iron, fiber, vitamins B_1, B_2, B_6, C, K and biotin, and have strong anti-aging and beautifying properties.

In Chinese medicine, carrots are said to be good for the health of the spleen, stomach and kidneys, and help eliminate excessive wind and cold out of the body. Check out the Beauty Detox recipes in Part III, as well as *The Beauty Detox Solution*, which offers creative ways to include more carrots in your diet.

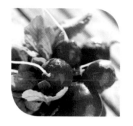

BEAUTY FOOD 26: RADISHES

Perhaps the only time you come in contact with the humble radish is when it's part of a plate of veggies and dip at a party or work function. Honestly, how often do you ever pick up and buy bunches of them at your grocery store? If you do, that's awesome, but most people don't. Nonetheless, radishes are easy to work into your diet, and I encourage you to start doing so because they're an exceptional hair-strengthening food, with plenty of vitamin C, as well as silicon and sulfur. Together, these elements help build healthy hair.

Professor Arnold Ehret cites radishes as a top mucus-dissolving food in *The Mucusless Diet Healing System*.[1] Radishes help cut and dissolve mucus in the digestive tract, so that nutrients can flow freely throughout the body to build beautiful hair. Radishes act as cleansers and detoxifiers, as do other members of the mustard family. The cleaner the body, the healthier the hair.

BEAUTY FOOD 27: NUTRITIONAL YEAST

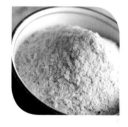

Nutritional yeast is the deactivated form of a primary yeast grown on a mixture of molasses and cane sugar. Don't let the word *yeast* scare you: there are various types of yeast, and while some are harmful, others are good. Nutritional yeast is gluten-free and is a different genus and species from the yeast that causes candidiasis, which is *Candida albicans*; nutritional yeast's biological classification is *Saccharomyces cerevisiae*. I've found even my clients who have candidiasis (see page 38) do well with it. Check it out at your local health food store.

Nutritional yeast contains the perfect combination of some of healthy hair's most important fuels: amino acids (protein) and B vitamins. It's an important component of my daily salads (see Kim's Classic Dressing in Part III). Nutritional yeast is a complete protein, with eighteen amino acids that will help fortify the protein in the hair shaft. Three tablespoons supply nine grams of complete protein, so adding it to recipes is an easy way to increase protein content. Because it is derived from a one-celled plant and its protein is easily absorbed from single amino acids, it generally combines well with most foods. On top of that it boasts fifteen key minerals, such as zinc, selenium, magnesium, manganese and copper.

One of the important hair benefits of nutritional yeast is that it's a rich source of the B-complex vitamins. With just three tablespoons, nutritional yeast provides more than the recommended daily value of most of the B vitamins, giving energy to your body's cells and keeping your hair's color strong and your hair shiny and healthy. It's also a rare plant-based source of B_{12}, which is important for nerve cell function among other important health functions (although supplementation of vitamin B_{12} for vegans is still generally recommended to ensure adequate absorption).

Nutritional yeast is naturally low in sodium and contains a high amount of fiber—about five grams per ounce. It contains a trace mineral, chromium, which is known as glucose tolerance factor (GTF). This is beneficial for helping to balance blood sugar levels. This, plus the hearty amount of protein, minerals and vitamins in nutritional yeast, makes it an exceptional hair, health and beauty food.

Recipes for Beautiful Hair

Roasted Portobello Mushroom and Creamy Dijon-Arugula Salad	207
Raw Curried Indian Veggies	284
Kim's Classic Dressing	188
Spinach-Basil Polenta with Creamy Sauce	276
Yin-Yang Meal: Baked Squash, Steamed Kale and Quinoa Pilaf	262
Spiralized Asian Veggie Salad	209
Kale, Carrot, Pinto Bean and Quinoa Stew	231
Kimberly's Kimchi	211
Quinoa Ten-Veggie "Fried Rice"	273
Green Spring Vegetable Risotto	254
Creamy Dijon-Tahini Dressing	190

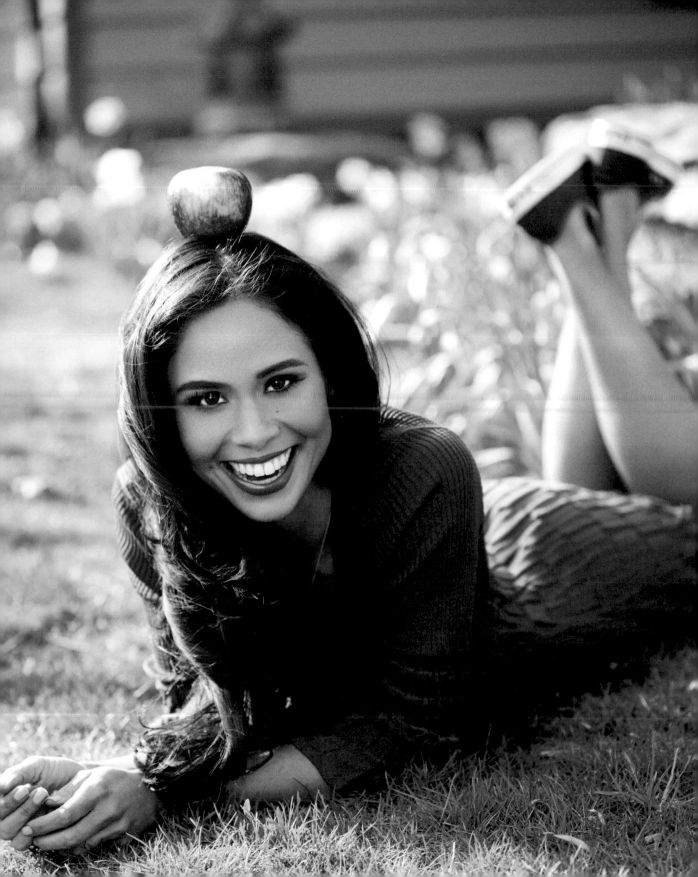

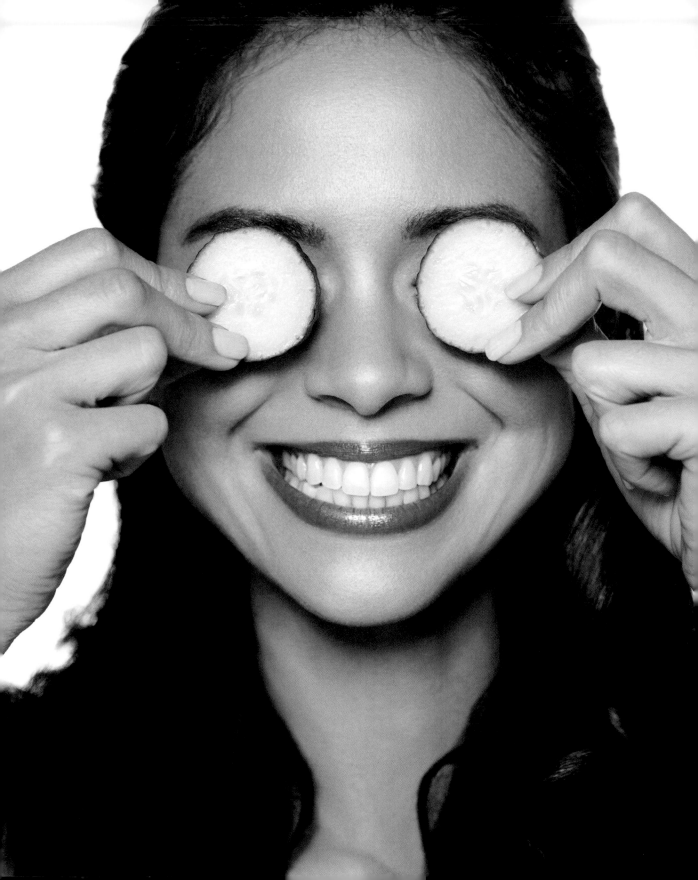

BEAUTIFUL EYES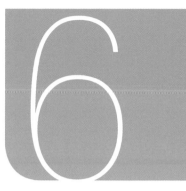

Women often define their own beauty by their skin and hair quality, but striking eyes are one of the most important and attractive qualities you can have. After all, when someone talks to you, he or she focuses on your eyes. Just as your other features can improve with your diet as you cleanse your body, the whites of your eyes can brighten, and your eye color can become more luminescent. Clear, sparkling eyes are reflective of inner health and abundant Beauty Energy . . . and are captivating.

BRIGHT EYES

There are countless nerve endings, tiny blood vessels and muscle fibers that are centered in the iris, and are linked to every part of the body. Signs of toxicity, congestion and ill health can lead to spots and irregularities around the pupil and iris.[1] Health practitioners in certain cultures around the world examine people's eyes to evaluate their health. Foods that are high in antioxidants, as well as foods that cleanse your system and flush out your lymphatic system, will banish cloudiness in your eyes and help you achieve beautiful, magnetic eyes.

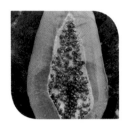

BEAUTY FOOD 28: PAPAYA

When I go to tropical places like Thailand and Puerto Rico . . . or New York City, I feast on papaya. Thankfully, it is pretty widely available nowadays, as other tropical fruit like bananas are. Papayas are high in the enzyme papain, which is similar to the stomach enzyme pepsin. It helps nourish and support the creation of beautiful eyes and healthy skin, by dissolving and cleansing old debris from the inside out and allowing nutrients to reach all areas of the body. In this way, papaya oxygenates the body and cleanses the tissues. The enzymes and vitamins in papaya help protect you against wrinkles and help alleviate existing damage, too.

Papayas help cleanse the body, soothe the digestive tract and promote digestion. They contain high concentrations of vitamins A and C, which repair the skin, keeping it youthful. Eating them often will help make your skin and hair's luster improve and make your skin more beautiful, while helping to brighten your eyes.

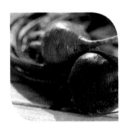

BEAUTY FOOD 29: BEETS

The beautiful red color of beets comes from the pigment betacyanin. It not only stimulates liver function, but is also absorbed into the blood corpuscles and helps oxygenate the blood, increasing the oxygen-carrying ability of the blood by up to 400 percent. The iron in beets makes them a powerful blood builder and cleanser, and pure blood transports nutrients better. Beets are a natural colon cleanser, removing toxins and congestion from the body, including from the capillaries traveling to the eye, so that your eyes can become brighter.

Beets are rich in antioxidants and calcium, iron, magnesium and fiber and have a high concentration of vitamins A and C. They're also filled with folate, which is key for new cell growth and healing.

Beets are extremely alkaline and high in antioxidants, making them a great balancer if you have an overly acidic condition. If you get them fresh at the farmers' market, be sure to take the green tops home with you and throw them in your Glowing Green Smoothie. Beet greens are one of the best leafy green sources for chlorophyll, iron, potassium and vitamins A and C.

Research has shown beets to be a potent anticancer and disease food, and helpful in normalizing blood pressure.[2] They may promote the elasticity of arteries, and, when consumed regularly, can help prevent varicose veins.

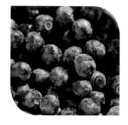

BEAUTY FOOD 30: BLUEBERRIES

Blueberries are a food that will make your eyes as well as skin beautiful. Their lovely blue color has to do with the antioxidant anthocyanin, which helps strengthen eyes and vision. Blueberries contain a special group of antioxidants called carotenoids and flavonoids; vitamins A, C and E; and selenium, zinc and phosphorus, which are all very beneficial and essential for eye health.

These powerhouse little berries have among the highest ORAC (oxygen radical absorbance capacity) scores of any food, meaning they have the highest levels of antioxidant capacity of all fresh fruits (acai's antioxidant level is higher, but it's only grown in South America, so it is flash-pasteurized and often distributed in a frozen form). The antioxidants work to destroy potentially aging free radicals better than almost any other food.

Blueberries also contain B vitamins (for energy), copper and iron. Blueberries are high in fiber, which provides roughage to the digestive tract, and blueberries are a relatively low-sugar fruit.

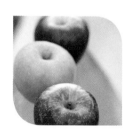

BEAUTY FOOD 31: APPLES

Clear, vivid eyes denote a clean, healthy body. Apples are a potent food to cleanse the body and give you those gorgeous eyes.

Pectin is the type of fiber found in apples, which makes up 75 percent of the apple's fiber. While other fruits also contain pectin, the highest concentration is found in apples. Pectin comes in both a soluble and an insoluble fiber form. The soluble form swells with water in the digestive tract, creating a gel-like substance that binds with fats in the intestine. This helps lower cholesterol and creates stable blood sugar levels. Apples' insoluble fiber is great roughage to keep you cleansing your colon efficiently. This contributes to clean blood and increased beauty, including health and beauty of the eyes. All this fiber is also very filling, so it acts as a natural way to control weight and calorie intake.

Apple pectin is a helpful detoxifier, as it has been reported to bind to and eliminate toxic metals from the body. It may help prevent DNA damage from free radicals by acting as an antioxidant. Researchers have found that the phytochemicals present in apple pectin may help decrease the risk of developing cardiovascular disease and strokes.[3]

Apple skin contains quercetin, an antioxidant compound that prevents damage to individual cells, including to the capillaries that supply nutrients around the body and to the eyes, and has potential protective effects against cancer.[4]

Most of the nutrition in apples is contained in its fiber and skin, so be sure to buy organic so you can consume the skins. These important benefits of the fiber in apples show how much better it is to not juice them, but instead eat them whole or include them in a whole form, like in the Glowing Green Smoothie. Green apples are lower in sugar than red apples, so if you have candidiasis (see Chapter 2) or are in the Blossoming Beauty Phase (see Chapter 3), use green Granny Smith apples, via the Glowing Green Smoothie, Low Sugar recipe (see Part III).

Recipes for Bright Eyes

ELIMINATING DARK CIRCLES AND PUFFINESS

When someone talks to you, they focus on your eyes. An even-toned, smooth eye area is beautiful, but puffiness and dark under-eye circles make you look tired, haggard and older. Although it's tempting to just slather on concealer to mask these issues, they never go away unless you get to the root cause. The good news is that you can learn to prevent and minimize dark circles and puffiness with your diet.

Dark circles are related to an overly taxed adrenal system. Excessive coffee, caffeine and refined sugars; lack of sleep; and stress all tax the adrenals. Another contributor may be when the blood vessels under the eyes get dilated and engorged, commonly caused by smoking and excessive salt intake. Dehydration may also be a factor, so be sure to drink plenty of fluids.

Puffiness can really show up in the under-eye skin area, which is very delicate and thin, and having too much sodium can make your eye area especially puff up. Cut out salty foods and cut back on your salt intake in general. Potassium helps flush out excess fluids from cells. Sticking to plant foods that naturally contain the proper balance of the electrolytes sodium to potassium in the first place can be helpful.

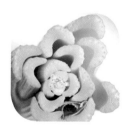

BEAUTY FOOD 32: CELERY

The balanced levels of potassium and sodium contained in celery can flush out excess bodily fluids, which can help reduce puffiness throughout the whole body and in the delicate under-eye area. It also has anti-inflammatory properties, as it contains a compound called polyacetylene.

Stress may also be a major contributor to dark under-eye circles. The father of medicine, Hippocrates, stated that celery has a calming effect on the nervous system, which may be attributed to its high concentration of organic alkaline minerals, including calcium, magnesium and potassium and because it helps lower high blood pressure. It contains compounds called pthalides that reduce stress hormones and relax the muscles around the arteries, which allows blood vessels to dilate.

A potent detoxifier, celery can help make the skin around the eyes (and the skin in general) look healthier. It aids the elimination of toxins from the body by promoting healthy and normal kidney function, which also helps to support the liver. Celery acts as a natural laxative. By now you know I'm a big fan of foods and cleansing methods that promote the elimination of wastes and toxins, which are one of the root causes of all your beauty concerns.

Look for celery with leaves attached to the stems, and don't throw them away. They have a high concentration of vitamin A, so toss them in with the celery stalks you include in your Glowing Green Smoothies and other recipes. The stalks are an excellent source of vitamins B_1, B_2, B_6 and C, and also contain folate and iron, plus essential amino acids.

BEAUTY FOOD 33: COLLARD GREENS

Collard greens are high in chlorophyll and the alkaline mineral magnesium, both of which can ease stress and help prevent you from overtaxing your adrenals, which can lead to dark under-eye circles.

Collards also provide a rich source of lipoic acid. This is a potent antioxidant to help regenerate vitamins C and E in the body, which assists in keeping your skin bright and healthy, and helps reduce discolorations and under-eye circles. Dark leafy greens such as collards contain the antioxidants lutein and xeaxanthan, which may be helpful in alleviating serious eye issues, such as macular degeneration.

Collards help brighten your overall skin tone. One cup of collard greens provides over 70 percent of the recommended daily allowance of vitamin C. Its high concentration of chlorophyll helps build healthy blood, which promotes better circulation and a healthy glow. Chlorophyll and human blood closely resemble each other on the molecular level, except chlorophyll contains magnesium while blood contains iron. Collards also contain high amounts of the skin- and hair-healthy vitamins A, B_1, B_2, B_6 and E. Collards are an excellent source of easily absorbable calcium, which, along with iron, keeps your blood vital and your bones strong.

There's a satisfying primal quality to eating whole collards. Their huge leaves remind me of jungle plants I saw in the Amazonian and Southeast Asian jungles that I visited on my round-the-world journey. Collards are thick, waxy leaves that look well equipped to sustain torrential rain forest downpours. Because they're so fibrous, be sure to chew them very well.

Research has revealed that certain phytonutrients present in collards and other cruciferous vegetables help eliminate toxins from the body by signaling genes to enhance the production of particular enzymes involved in the process of detoxification. Collard greens are nature's natural ingredient to create wraps. Replacing flour and corn tortillas with them is one of the easiest ways to work them into your diet. You'll find they make a satisfying wrap that also increases your beauty.

BEAUTY FOOD 34: ASPARAGUS

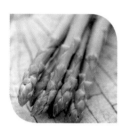

Puffy circles in the thin, delicate under-eye area may often be the result of an overdose of sodium. Per cup, asparagus has 288 milligrams of potassium and is very low in sodium, which means that eating asparagus helps create the proper electrolyte balance in the body and reduces puffiness and bloating. Asparagus is also high in fiber, which cleanses the digestive tract and supports ongoing detoxification efforts.

Asparagus contains vitamin A and is a plant-based source of glutathione, an antioxidant that helps scavenge free radicals. Both of these compounds help your skin stay healthy and youthful overall. Asparagus is also one of the best sources of vitamin K, which helps the body absorb calcium, thus promoting proper bone formation and repair.

Because of its strong detoxifying properties, asparagus has been shown to help prevent and treat urinary tract infections and kidney stones.

BEAUTY FOOD 35: BANANAS

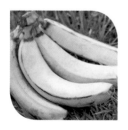

Lack of beauty sleep is a big contributor to dark under-eye circles, and bananas are rich in vitamin B_6, which helps ward off irritability and insomnia, as well as magnesium, which promotes better sleep patterns. Research also shows that the combination of nutrients, healthy carbs and the essential amino acid tryptophan in bananas can fight depression and help you stay in a good mood. This is helpful for skin health, because when you're happy, you tend to sleep and eat better and make better lifestyle choices.

Bananas have a high concentration of fiber and ascorbic acid (vitamin C), which helps promote good digestion and prevents constipation. They contribute to healthy blood pressure and cholesterol levels, and help keep adrenal-taxing anxiety in check. Bananas are a plentiful source of potassium, which helps regulate proper fluid levels in the body. Its vitamin A and natural oils also help keep the skin moisturized. I have to say that bananas certainly make me happy, and as they are one of my favorite foods in the world, I sure do eat a lot of them.

Bananas grow abundantly in many areas of the world and are a rich source of vitamins and minerals. Because they have a wonderfully sweet taste, they can help satisfy sweet cravings in the diet so you don't have to resort to processed sugary treats high in fat.

Be sure to eat ripe bananas that are yellow with black spots, because when bananas are ripe, they're more alkaline-forming. Store bananas on the counter to ripen. If you have too many ripe bananas at once, you can peel and freeze them. They're great to use in your Glowing Green Smoothie.

Recipes for Eliminating Dark Circles and Puffiness

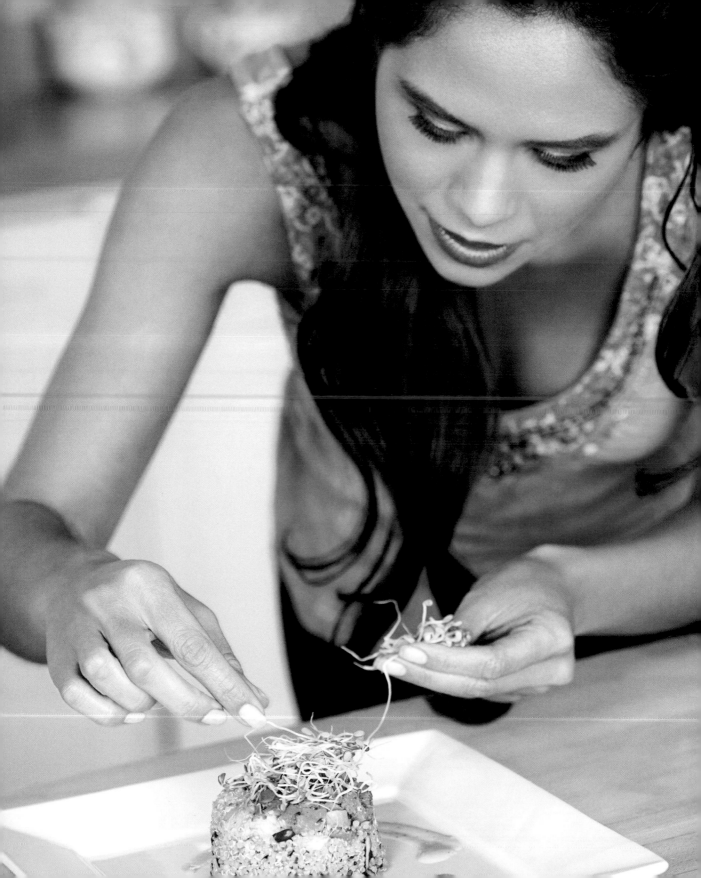

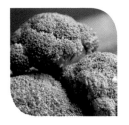

BEAUTY FOOD 36: BROCCOLI

Broccoli is a grace-inspiring beauty food that nourishes not only the skin, but also the joints and connective tissue around the body to help you move fluidly. Because it's high in such an array of beauty minerals, including calcium, magnesium and zinc, broccoli helps keep your bones strong, and also keeps your body more alkaline. When your body is more alkaline, you retain calcium better in your bones. It's leached out of your bones when you consume acidic products, like dairy and soda. Another great feature, especially for women, is broccoli's high concentration of folate and iron, which keeps the blood healthy, the circulation flowing and anemia at bay. Iron's absorption is optimized in the presence of vitamin C, and because broccoli has both, it's an ideal combination. Broccoli helps prevent movement issues associated with aging, like osteoporosis and arthritis, keeping you moving youthfully and gracefully.

Broccoli contains vitamin A, which has collagen-smoothing and repairing properties, as well as the important beauty minerals iron, calcium, zinc, magnesium, potassium and chromium. It is also full of phytonutrients and antioxidants.

Broccoli has fabulous anti-aging benefits, as it is full of phytonutrients, fiber and antioxidants, making it effective at neutralizing free radicals and helping to purge the body of toxins. Broccoli also contains a compound called sulforaphane, which may alleviate inflammation and skin damage from the sun.

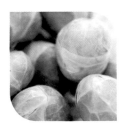

BEAUTY FOOD 37: BRUSSELS SPROUTS

Your body's detox system requires an ample supply of sulfur to function optimally, and Brussels sprouts are rich in sulfur-containing nutrients. Brussels sprouts are an outstanding source of glucosinolates, which create detox-activated compounds called isothiocyanates. Recent studies have shown that certain compounds in Brussels sprouts block the activity of sulphotransferase enzymes that can be detrimental to the health and stability of DNA within white blood cells.[1]

To further fight toxicity in the body and keep you moving well, Brussels sprouts are an excellent source of vitamins A, C and E, as well as the antioxidant mineral manganese. Brussels sprouts contain vitamin K, which provides anti-inflammatory properties that help keep joints healthy and moving gracefully, as well as a wide variety of antioxidant phytonutrients, including many antioxidant flavonoids. In fact, one study in France examined the total intake of antioxidant polyphenols and found Brussels sprouts to be a more important dietary contributor to these antioxidants than any other cruciferous vegetable, including broccoli.[2]

Although this may sound surprising, Brussels sprouts contain a good dose of omega-3 fatty acids. About one-and-a-half cups contain more than one-third of the daily ALA amount included in the National Academy of Sciences' Dietary Reference Intake recommendations. Brussels sprouts are also a good source of calcium, important for healthy bone formation and maintenance, which is critical to being able to move fluidly, as well as potassium and folate. One-quarter of the calories in Brussels sprouts are from protein. Being high in fiber, too, Brussels sprouts can help lower cholesterol by binding with bile acids that are produced from cholesterol in the liver and carry them out of the body as waste. The more bile acids are removed, the more the body pulls cholesterol from the bloodstream, which is necessary to produce more bile salts, thereby helping to increase the excretion of cholesterol from the body.

Brussels sprouts can be eaten raw (check out the raw Brussels Sprout Salad in Part III), to benefit from the full level of vitamin content, but are also beneficial cooked: cut them into quarters and steam them for a few minutes, then add any dressing. Delish!

BEAUTY FOOD 38: SESAME SEEDS

Sesame seeds are an ancient seed (remember the old "Open Sesame!" saying from the *Tales of the Arabian Nights* stories when you were a kid? When I was traveling in Morocco I had flashbacks of this favorite childhood book of mine.) and are among the most concentrated plant-based sources of calcium.

Sesame seeds are also high in other important minerals—including iron, zinc, magnesium, manganese and copper—that have roles in maintaining bodily structure, bone mineralization, red blood cell production and enzyme synthesis. They're also a good source of B-complex vitamins, such as niacin, folate, thiamin, pyridoxine and riboflavin, as well as fiber.

Copper is an important trace mineral that has numerous anti-inflammatory qualities and plays a role in antioxidant enzyme systems. Copper also figures prominently in the activity of lysyl oxidase, an enzyme that supports collagen and elastin, the compounds that your body needs to provide elasticity and strength to your bones, joints, blood vessels and skin.

Sesame seeds contain two unique fiber compounds, called sesamin and sesamolin. Among other benefits, these have been shown to fight free radical damage, help prevent high blood pressure and increase vitamin E supplies in animals. Sesamin has also been found to protect the liver from oxidative damage.

Sesame seeds are a good source of high-quality dietary protein. The seeds are also especially rich in the monounsaturated fatty acid called oleic acid.

Sesame seeds contain natural oil, so it's important to keep them tightly covered and ideally stored in the refrigerator to ensure that they stay fresh and resist rancidity. Sesame oil is one of the few oils I use in small amounts, as it adds a wonderful flavor to dishes. Tahini is a paste made of ground sesame seeds, which is a component of my raw chickpea-less hummus recipe in *The Beauty Detox Solution*, and in Creamy Dijon-Tahini Dressing in Part III of this book. Always choose raw tahini, if it's available.

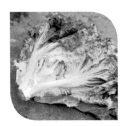

BEAUTY FOOD 39: ROMAINE LETTUCE

Romaine lettuce has always been a favorite green of mine. It is terrifically rich in nutrients, and shouldn't be confused with its sickly relative, iceberg lettuce, which is virtually nutrient-free.

Moving fluidly and gracefully has a lot to do with antioxidants, which help eliminate free radicals that contribute to aging and deterioration of all your body parts. Romaine lettuce is a fibrous leafy green, and contains lots of vitamin C and beta-carotene, which converts to vitamin A in the body. Vitamin C and beta-carotene work together to keep cholesterol from oxidizing, which is important in preventing plaque from forming in artery walls. It is also a rich source of folate and potassium, which help regulate blood pressure. Romaine lettuce is a good source of iron, which, combined with the vitamin C it contains for enhanced absorption, makes it a great blood builder to help with graceful movement. Romaine contains a high concentration of water, and is also rich in vitamin K, manganese, vitamins B_1 and B_2, chromium and other minerals like molybdenum.

Romaine truly is a super-versatile green, with broad, dark-green leaves that can be used in everything from salads to roll-ups and wraps. With such a high nutrient content and mild taste, romaine is a staple ingredient in the Glowing Green Smoothie. Also check out my recipe in Part III for Raw Vegan Caesar Salad, a healthy twist on the romaine lettuce-centered classic.

CELLULITE-FREE BODY

Cellulite is fat that pushes through the skin's collagen to form wrinkles and bumps. You may not be able to magically get rid of all cellulite with a few special foods, but if you keep your body toned and lower in fat overall, you may be able to reduce the visibility and amount of cellulite in your body.

Another aspect of cellulite is why it's so visible in the first place. When fat starts to poke up through the collagen in the skin, the collagen may lack optimal connective tissue structure to support a smooth, undimpled shape.[3] Genetics may play a role here, but so can the foods you eat: those that contain nutrients to support collagen or foods that weaken collagen by causing inflammation may cause the breakdown of collagen and elastin and make skin age faster. You can make your collagen more resilient by eating many of the collagen-strengthening and anti-inflammatory nutrients contained in all the beauty foods throughout this section.

Because acidic toxins and wastes tend to be stored in your fat cells, reducing toxins in your body helps your body rid itself of stored fat, and can therefore help with cellulite. The body stores these toxins and wastes in fat cells to keep the toxins intact and away from the vital organs. When your body's pH becomes more alkaline (see Chapter 2), your body tends to allow these toxins to be expelled from your body, and your fat cells may shrink, making cellulite less visible. Ways you can make your body more alkaline include consuming more alkaline-forming foods, especially fresh greens and other vegetables and fruit, avoiding smoking and polluted environments as much as possible, and using natural cleaning and body care products. Avoiding particularly acid-forming foods, such as sodas, artificial sweeteners and preservatives, dairy, and excessively consuming animal products, will also help balance your body's pH. Regular exercise is important for general health and will help, but remember that in general the way your body looks is more strongly affected by the food you eat, even more than the exercise you do.

The Glowing Green Smoothie: Long-Term Fat-Burner

The Glowing Green Smoothie (see page 168 for the recipe) is one of the easiest and tastiest ways to drink your beauty foods. It is an amazing long-term fat-burner because it combines fresh fruit and vegetables with a bevy of fiber, phytonutrients, minerals, vitamins and enzymes that help flush out the pollutants and toxins stored in your fat cells. The large amounts of greens you're getting in this one smoothie are blended, so they're very easy for your body to absorb. You can get more greens with this one smoothie than several salads put together (and without having to use any dressing), and this smoothie is incredibly alkalizing. All my clients love the GGS—and virtually all of them say it's changed their lives! On www.kimberlysnyder.net, you can read reviews from actual members who discuss their GGS experiences.

BEAUTY FOOD 40: FRESH CILANTRO AND PARSLEY

The fresh herbs of parsley and cilantro are associated with cleansing characteristics, by removing heavy metals from the body (also called chelation) that lodge in and enlarge the fat cells.[4] This chelation process can be significant in preventing aging, because heavy metals can disrupt normal tissue function and may be the source of millions of free radicals in the tissues of the body. Upon removing heavy metals, the tissues can begin to heal and function normally.

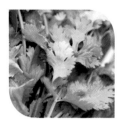

Cilantro

Cilantro has been shown in experiments to help chelate mercury from the body. Dr. Yoshiaki Omura, director of medical research of the Heart Disease Research Foundation and president of the International College of Acupuncture in New York, headed up some of this research by showing that after heavy mercury exposure, eating cilantro could lead to the excretion of mercury through the urine.[5] Dr. Omura also discovered that his patients had fewer colds and flu after removing the heavy metals, because it appears that viruses and bacteria like to congregate in organs contaminated by heavy metals. Another researcher, Dietrich Klinghardt, M.D., Ph.D., recommends cilantro as one of the best means to remove mercury from the brain.[6] This is especially useful to note for fish and seafood eaters, who may unknowingly consume much more mercury than they realize. The researchers also found that cilantro accelerated the elimination of mercury, lead and aluminum through the urine.[7]

Cilantro, also called Chinese parsley, is an optional ingredient in the Glowing Green Smoothie recipe for these very metal-cleansing properties. Note that chlorella, also discussed in Chapter 8, is also said to be a wonderful aid in binding and excreting heavy metals.

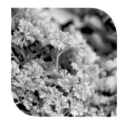

Parsley

It's a real shame some people think of parsley as a garnish. It's so much more than a pretty decoration. Parsley has been credited in holistic health for being a potent detoxifier and diuretic, helping to prevent bloating and water retention by flushing out the kidneys.[8]

It is widely known as an aid to digestion, a help in removing toxins from the body, and a blood cleanser and purifier. Parsley, rich in vitamins A, C and E, plus minerals, is a powerful antioxidant. For all these reasons, parsley is a great anticellulite food. Parsley is also a good source of folate and is rich in iron, to help maintain your healthy glow. I incorporate it often into my Glowing Green Smoothie.

BEAUTY FOOD 41: BUCKWHEAT AND OAT GROATS

I include both buckwheat and oat groats in this section on cellulite because these two foods are slow-burning, easily digestible forms of fuel that contain important nutrients, such as B vitamins, protein and fiber. They'll help keep you full and satisfied, which will prevent you from snacking on fattening foods. They're both really high in fiber, which is key in a long-term anticellulite program: fiber helps move and clear out toxins that will become released from fat cells, so that they don't recirculate throughout the body. Using buckwheat and oat groats is a natural way to replace commercial cereals and granola, and they are more nutritious foods than those products. Both are gluten-free and easy to digest, especially when they're soaked (or, in the case of buckwheat, both soaked and sprouted).

Buckwheat

Buckwheat is a complete protein that contains all essential amino acids, along with essential fatty acids. It's high in the amino acid lysine, which is great for tissue repair and can be helpful in repairing collagen. What's more, one-quarter cup of dried buckwheat groats contains five grams of fiber as well as six grams of protein. It's high in many of the B vitamins, as well as phosphorus, magnesium (which helps relax the mind and balance the levels of other nutrients, such as calcium, in your body), iron, folate, zinc, copper, and manganese (one cup supplies 25 percent of the daily value of manganese), as well as flavonoids.

Buckwheat is also a complex, whole grain so it's great for diabetes patients and those with hypoglycemia, who need help stabilizing blood sugar levels. Buckwheat has also been found to lower blood pressure and cholesterol.

Other Ways to Enjoy Buckwheat

Kasha, the cooked form of buckwheat, is also beneficial, although I prefer preparing buckwheat raw and sprouted. Buckwheat flour is a beneficial, key ingredient in my Buckwheat Gluten-Free Vegan Pancakes recipe in Part III on page 179. Soba noodles are made from buckwheat, and are a great alternative to wheat; an entrée I often order at a Japanese restaurant is a huge bowl of soup with vegetables and soba noodles.

Oat Groats

Just as millet shouldn't be just for birds, oats aren't just for horses. Up to 95 percent of oats produced worldwide are for consumption by horses, leaving a mere 5 percent for human consumption. Yet oats are another high-nutrient plant food that has a full spectrum of nutrition, including vitamin E, B vitamins and minerals (calcium, magnesium, potassium, selenium, copper, zinc, iron and manganese).

Oats contain both soluble and insoluble fiber, making them quite filling; they also don't spike your blood sugar the way refined carbohydrates and sugars do. In a study at Harvard School of Public Health in Boston, it was determined that consumption of whole grains can contribute to favorable metabolic alterations that may reduce long-term weight gain.[8] This, along with fat reduction, will help reduce cellulite.

In studies at the University of Kentucky, a whole-grain, bean, vegetable and fruit–rich diet enabled type 1 diabetes patients (who don't produce any insulin themselves) to cut their daily insulin intake by 38 percent.[9] Oats have been found to benefit heart health, lower blood pressure levels[10, 11, 12] and can even help prevent diabetes as part of a high whole-grain diet.

I recommend oat groats, which are the most natural, unprocessed form of oats, but if you have trouble finding them at your local grocery or health food market you can get steel-cut oats (also called Irish oatmeal), which are the groats cut into pieces with a steel cutter. While naturally gluten-free, to prevent cross-contamination with gluten, choose oats that are organic and have been processed in a gluten-free facility. In Part III and in *The Beauty Detox Solution,* I include a recipe for Raw Rolled Oat Cereal, but cooking oats is also good. Just be sure to avoid processed, instant oatmeal, which often has additives such as salt, sugar and artificial sweeteners.

OTHER GOOD CELLULITE FOODS

A diet high in essential fatty acids and antioxidant minerals will help regulate your body's fat metabolism. Nuts and seeds are good selections in this category. All citrus fruits, too, are especially useful in ridding yourself of cellulite by providing your body with a big boost of vitamin C to rebuild and repair skin collagen, which prevents cellulite from being so visible. Lemons are a terrific choice, as are grapefruit and oranges.

TONED BODY

Just as beauty implies health, so does strength. A strong, beautiful body is healthy and incredibly attractive. No one wants an excess of fat, but a stick-thin, overly skinny body lacks the visceral power to perform many of life's important tasks, and can make you less attractive to the opposite sex as a potential good mate. Neither too fat nor too thin, a toned body radiates magnetic energy and is incredibly sexy. Exercise helps, but the right foods on which to build muscle, regenerate cells and improve tone are also critical. I used to spend a great deal more time working out, but now I don't ever really "work out" per se—at least not in the traditional sense. I'm not a gym person. But I am a vinyasa yoga junkie, and I like to practice four to five times a week (depending on if my crazy schedule allows). Yoga has the added benefit of encouraging deep breathing and bringing oxygen throughout the body. I also stay active with lots of walking and hiking when I'm in a place that I can.

The great news is that my body looks more toned than ever before, thanks to the Beauty Detox program. This is especially true for my arms, which I used to always wish would actually show more muscle tone! I'm excited for you, too, to personally experience that an alkaline-rich diet and continuous cleansing allow for more oxygen to circulate to your muscles, and will help your body look more toned overall as well.

How Exercise Fits In

Cardiovascular exercise is an important part of any beauty regimen, as it brings oxygen to the tissues and muscles, and helps to cleanse out wastes and acids. Some form of weight-bearing exercise is important for maintaining bone health as well. Find the exercise that most appeals to you. Why not try something fun, like a salsa dance class or paddle boarding? The more fun you have working out and staying active, the more likely you'll keep it up on a regular and long-term basis.

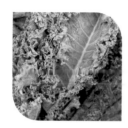

BEAUTY FOOD 42: KALE

Kale is a major strengthening food for your body—you can tell just from looking at its super-hardy, waxy leaves. Kale comes in several varieties, but my personal favorite is the deep forest green–colored Lacinato kale, also known as dinosaur or Italian kale. Kale is at the very top of my list of foods that have had the most impact on my personal health and beauty. I learned about its powers at a yoga studio in New York City, where many of my fellow yoga students, both men and women, ate copious amounts of kale on a weekly basis, practiced lots of yoga, and were incredibly toned and muscled. When I started doing the same thing (along with incorporating the other important eating and cleansing principles mentioned in Part I), I noticed a big change in my body: I started seeing muscles in places throughout my arms and back where I never used to be toned. I was wowed that it was possible to see those muscles without weight lifting. Today, I consume kale as a large part of my dinner at least several times a week.

Like other dark, leafy greens, kale provides a superior source of free-form amino acids, which are singular molecules that are not attached by peptide bonds to other amino acids, and can be assimilated directly into the body and built into protein. It also contains large amounts of manganese, iron, copper and calcium.

As an anti-aging tool, kale wages a powerful battle on free radicals and cellular oxidation by supplying copious amounts of the powerful antioxidants known as carotenoids and flavonoids, which protect your cells from free radicals that cause oxidative stress. The key flavonoids kaempferol and quercitin (not to mention the forty-five other distinctive flavonoids in kale), have also been shown to specifically fight against the formation of cancerous cells. For these reasons, along with its high levels of vitamins A and C, kale helps keep your body strong and resilient.

Although you may not usually think of greens as supplying healthy fats, one cup of kale provides about 10 percent of the RDA of omega-3 fatty acids, which help regulate hormones in your body and offer anti-inflammatory properties. Kale also has a high level of vitamin K, which helps fight the anti-inflammation battle and protects against stiff joints and arthritis. Kale's high level of vitamin K works with calcium and supports the processes necessary to build strong bones.

High in fiber, kale also helps make sure you're properly expelling wastes and toxins from your body. The other way it helps with detoxification is by means of the isothiocyanates (ITC) from glucosinolates it contains, which aid in the body's detoxification. Kale contains sulforaphane, which encourages the liver to produce enzymes that detoxify cancer-causing chemicals. Yes, kale is a good friend to us in many ways.

BEAUTY FOOD 43: HEMP SEEDS

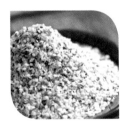

Hemp is one of the best foods to build long, lean muscle tone. Hemp supplies a rich source of easily assimilated amino acids, including the essential amino acids your body can't produce. These will provide strong building blocks to boost your muscle tone, as well as the proteins necessary for vibrant skin, hair and nails.

Hemp possesses one of nature's most concentrated plant sources of essential fatty acids (even greater than the mighty flaxseed), while exhibiting the perfect ratio of three-to-one omega-6 linoleic acid to omega-3 linoleic acid. It is truly a super-seed, loaded with phytonutrients to nourish healthy blood, tissues, cells and organs that make for a beautiful, toned body. Hemp also provides a rich array of minerals, including zinc, calcium, magnesium and iron.

Three tablespoons of hemp seeds supply eleven grams of easily assimilated protein. If you're looking to build bulkier muscle and add additional protein to your diet, one of the best ways to do that is through a hemp protein shake—combined with heavier lifting exercises. Check out the Power Protein Smoothie in Part III on page 173.

Hemp is a superior plant protein and when used in shakes will not cause bloating or gas (signs of poorly digesting foods), which is frequently the case with whey and other processed proteins. Soy protein is also a poor choice for many reasons (more on this in Chapter 2); among other faults, it contains very high amounts of phytic acid, which prevents you from absorbing minerals. Hemp seeds don't contain phytic acid. Raw protein powders derived from brown rice, sprouts and other non-soy plant foods are also good choices.

And don't worry, in case it crossed your mind: this variety of hemp seeds will certainly not give you the drug high of marijuana, which contains an extremely concentrated form of THC. You'd have to consume pounds of hemp seeds in one sitting to even mildly feel anything. So, no laughing fits or munchies.

I love that hemp seeds are a global health food. They have been consumed around the world, from China, Russia and the Sotho tribe in southern Africa to Poland and Lithuania, where the people make a hemp seed soup called *semieniatka.*

Hemp seeds contain an especially beneficial type of omega-6 fat called gamma-linolenic acid (GLA). GLA can help support a healthy metabolism and fat-burning functions, which will also help you achieve and maintain a toned body. It is also useful in balancing hormones; supporting the health of skin, hair and nails; and offering anti-inflammatory properties. GLA is not commonly found in many foods, but making hemp seeds a regular part of your diet will ensure you're getting a good amount in your diet. I sprinkle hemp seeds whole on salads, and enjoy the Power Protein Smoothie regularly.

BEAUTY FOOD 44: QUINOA

Quinoa is an ancient grain that has been cultivated in the Andean mountain areas of South America for over five thousand years. The Incas believed quinoa was a sacred food, and referred to it as *chisaya mama,* or the "mother of all grains." I ate it often when I was backpacking through Peru, and it became a godsend for me, as I didn't partake in the guinea pig, fried eggs and white bread that were ubiquitous there.

Quinoa supplies one of the most nutritious forms of complex carbs in the world, which are necessary for building muscle and a toned body. But while some grains just provide carbs, quinoa will feed your body so much more. It is a great source of complete plant protein that contains all essential amino acids the body requires as the building blocks for muscle. As a grain, it is still classified and combines as a starch, however, and though it contains amino acids, it is not a dense protein like animal protein, which contains long amino acid chains that need to be broken down upon digestion. It is especially abundant in the amino acid lysine, essential for tissue growth and repair.

Compared to other grains, such as wheat, quinoa is higher in minerals, including calcium, phosphorus, magnesium, potassium, iron, zinc and the antioxidant minerals copper and manganese, as well as other phytonutrients. Quinoa contains high levels of magnesium, which helps relax the blood vessels and muscles.

Quinoa is rich in fiber, which helps ensure elimination of toxins and keeps your digestive tract cleansed—an important factor in a toned body. Pooping is good! Because quinoa is gluten-free, it's a perfect grain for Blossoming Beauties (see Chapter 3) as well as any other Beauty Detox phase. As with all grains, be sure to eat a large green salad beforehand, and have cooked or raw veggies along with it to serve as a natural form of portion restriction.

Help for Migraine Headaches

Quinoa and millet both contain high levels of magnesium, which has been shown to help relax blood vessels and prevent constriction that can contribute to migraines. Riboflavin (also called vitamin B_2), which is also found in these grains, is necessary for proper energy production within cells. Riboflavin has been shown to reduce the frequency of attacks in migraine sufferers, most likely by bolstering the energy metabolism within brain and muscle cells.

BEAUTY FOOD 45: MILLET

The thing I've always found funny about millet, which is technically a seed, is that people throw millet to the birds in a birdfeeder, while feeding themselves foods that are inferior in nutrition. But it's not a bird food in much of the world. Millet is said to have originally been cultivated ten thousand years ago in East Asia, and has since been consumed for thousands of years across Africa, China, India, Greece and Egypt.

Millet is one of the few grains that is alkaline-forming in the body, is gluten-free, is easily digested by almost everyone and is nutritious and packed with minerals, making it one of the top Beauty Detox grains.

Millet is a remarkable source of plant-based protein combined with complex carbohydrates, both of which are important for building a beautifully toned body (like quinoa, it is classified as a starch, though it contains easily assimilated amino acids). It is also a good source of vitamin B$_1$, which supports muscles and a healthy nervous system, among other functions. The phosphorus in millet aids in fat metabolism, body tissue repair and the creation of energy, as phosphorus is an essential component of ATP (*adenosine triphosphate*), which is a nucleotide that is a major source of energy for metabolic processes.

Packed with fiber and so many phytonutrients, millet is an all-around power food. Other important nutrients it contains are calcium, manganese, tryptophan and phosphorus, most of the B vitamins, vitamins E and K, iron, zinc, copper and omega-3 fatty acids. Its manganese content helps build strong, healthy bones and a healthy thyroid gland, which regulates your metabolism and may help maintain hair color. Millet also calms and soothes the nerves by supplying serotonin to the body.

Millet is also a rich source of magnesium, which acts as a cofactor in a number of enzymatic reactions in the body, regulating the secretion of glucose and insulin (see the "Help for Migraine Headaches" sidebar).

I cook millet regularly and serve it to my clients. Use it interchangeably with quinoa, because it, too, is gluten-free. Millet bread is now fairly easy to find in the frozen section of grocery stores. Check out my Spanish Millet Paella recipe in Part III on page 245.

BEAUTY FOOD 46: CHIA SEEDS

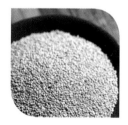

Over the years, chia seeds have grown so much in importance in my own diet that they're now the most plentiful seed I consume on a regular basis. I consider chia seeds one of the most important foods to maintain the tone of my body and my health in general. I also use them in smoothies that I give my clients to keep them lean and strong.

Chia seeds swell to ten to fifteen times their original size when exposed to liquid, forming a gel, which helps you stay full for hours. The ancient Aztec warriors consumed chia seeds during their conquests and long runs to help increase their stamina and endurance. They make an excellent workout food for you as well, while supplying your body with strengthening and toning nutrients. I consume them after yoga classes and during long hikes.

Because they have such a high level of both soluble and insoluble fiber, chia seeds promote a slow conversion of starches into sugars in your body, which helps balance blood sugar levels, so they help keep your energy steady for hours and throughout your workout, and also help replace amino acids after a workout.

To further contribute to a toned body, chia is a complete protein: it contains all essential amino acids, to repair the muscle tissue in your body and keep you looking more toned, while raising energy levels. Because of their combination of protein, vitamins, minerals and fibrous gel, chia seeds supply you with a steady, long-burning source of energy that is also extremely helpful in ensuring that you don't excessively snack on less-than-optimal food that would hinder your weight goals.

Chia seeds also help with ongoing cleansing. Their fibrous, gelatinous material promotes optimal digestion, keeping your colon hydrated and making sure that foods move easily through your system so that waste, which can end up being stored in fat cells, is reduced. Their outer shell is easily broken upon consumption, so you don't have to grind them up like flaxseeds to absorb the nutrients.

Chia seeds provide an extremely rich plant source of omega-3 fatty acids, without all the pollution and serious toxin concerns of consuming fish (though an algae-based DHA supplement can be good nutritional insurance; see Part I). The word *chia* is derived from a word in the South American Nahuatl language that means "oily." Chia oil contains about 64 percent concentrated omega-3 fatty acids, which are important for hormonal balance, nerve function and so many other functions.

Chia seeds are extremely high in antioxidants, which help them stay fresh at room temperature for two years without any preservatives, unlike flaxseeds, which go rancid much more easily. These antioxidants help eliminate aging free radicals, which are created from a polluted environment and poor dietary choices, as well as oxidative stress from intense, extended workouts.

By consuming chia seeds, you'll not only be getting calcium, but also the bone-important minerals magnesium and boron, which enable calcium to be absorbed. Need I say more? As you can see from this very long list of benefits, chia seeds are one of my favorite Beauty Foods.

Recipes for a Toned Body

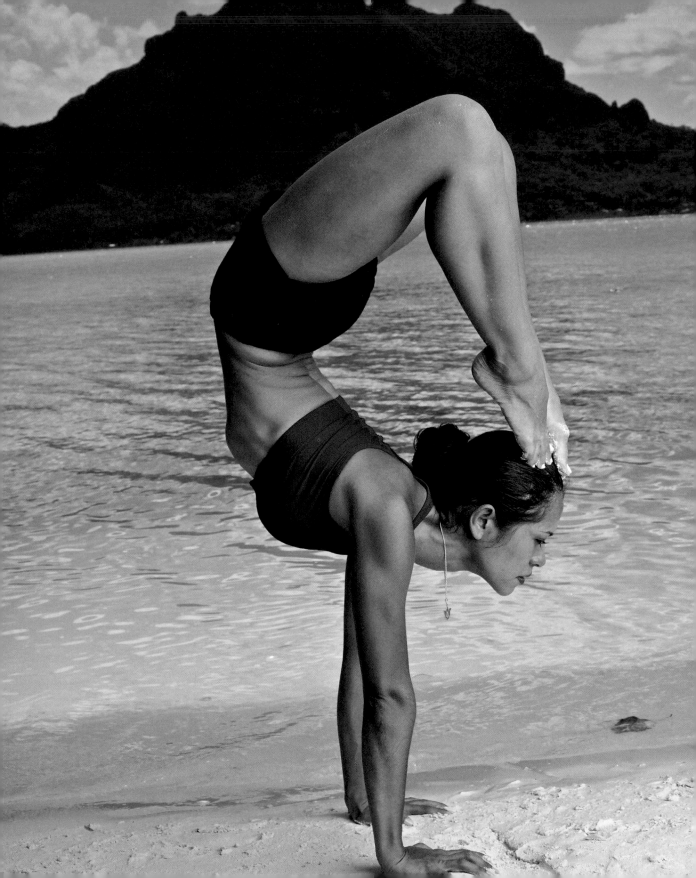

INNER GLOW 8

True beauty can never be derived from pills and products alone. Even if you don't have the most perfect features or hair, a magnetic inner glow can make you even more attractive than people who have such features. The glow extends not only to your physical appearance, but also to your overall energy and radiance.

BEAUTY FOOD 47: BEE POLLEN

Abundantly overflowing with vitamins, minerals and enzymes, bee pollen will enhance your overall glow, beauty and energy. Just look at the bees themselves and their incessant activity (bzzz). Bees are amazing, energized beings that can visit up to several thousand flowers a day.

Bee pollen allows you to ingest the extremely rich nutrition product of their hours of energy. Each bee pollen granule contains around four million pollen grains, and one teaspoon of pollen contains anywhere from two to ten billion pollen grains, which have the ability to fertilize flowers and other plants.[1]

Said to have been consumed by the Chinese for centuries to help increase energy, fight acne and depression, and improve digestion, bee pollen is also associated with improved fertility and libido, which make you attractive to the opposite sex.

Filled with all the B vitamins (except B_{12}), bee pollen provides stress relief, improves digestion and balances your hormones, while assisting in cleansing toxins from the body. Bee pollen contains rutin (an enzyme catalyst), potent antioxidants, all essential amino acids, essential fatty acids and nucleic acids, such as RNA and DNA.

Bee pollen has high levels of collagen-repairing vitamin C and skin-protecting vitamin E, making it a potent anti-aging, antiwrinkle food. Ingesting these nutrients provides an internal form of sun protection, guarding you against harmful UV rays that create skin-damaging free radicals. Packed with living enzymes, bee pollen also assists your body in digesting and optimally absorbing nutrition from other foods you consume.

One of the richest sources of complete protein in nature, bee pollen comes in a form that's readily available to the body. Bee pollen supplies concentrated complete protein to the body with all essential amino acids, including the amino acid phenylalanine, which helps to control hunger and appetite. I've found that consuming bee pollen is so nutritionally complete that it helps you eat less food overall and also balances cravings. Some researchers believe bee pollen helps improve metabolism and weight loss efforts. Bee pollen naturally comprises 15 percent lecithin, which is thought to protect the nervous system and brain against radiation and some environmental contaminants,[2] and promotes the elimination of fat stores from the body.

Bee pollen further provides a rich source of beauty minerals, including calcium, iron, potassium and zinc. (A deficiency of zinc may contribute to acne.) There have been some anecdotal reports that bee pollen has been helpful in alleviating eczema and psoriasis.

It is crucial that you obtain bee pollen from an environmentally healthy region and from an ethical beekeeper to ensure that the bees are treated well, the nutrients mentioned here are fully supplied and the facilities and regions for harvesting are free from heavy pollution. Heavy pollution and overpopulation can lead to a compromised environment, which, in turn, compromises the bee pollen. If the environment is full of heavy metals, like lead and airborne chemicals, for example, they can contaminate the pollen.

Bee pollen helps increase your stamina, energy and immunity.[3] I often take a tablespoon of bee pollen before going to yoga or as a quick snack on the go. If you're chronically fatigued, which is the opposite of glowing, bee pollen may help you improve your energy levels.

Note that if you have a known or suspected pollen or bee allergy, you should probably avoid bee pollen (though it isn't produced in the body of the bee). Start with a very small amount if you're new to consuming bee pollen—approximately one quarter of a teaspoon—and build up from there. I try to have about one tablespoon a day, or at least a few times a week. You can commonly find bee pollen in the refrigerated section of any health food store, but if you can find a local, organic bee farm, that would be even better. It's always a treat for me to visit my beekeeper and his beehives on his organically farmed land, where he handles the bees lovingly with his bare hands (the bees never sting him), to source the freshest pollen for me and my clients. The bee pollen we use at GLOW Bio, my organic smoothie and juice shops, is sourced from my beekeeper.

BEAUTY FOOD 48: SUNFLOWER SEEDS

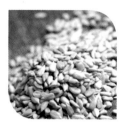

Because they are derived from the beautiful sunflower, ever turned to the sun, it's easy to see how sunflower seeds impart glowing qualities. Natural health advocate Ann Wigmore includes sunflower seed cheese and sprouts as daily staples of her program. Her research revealed the sunflower seed to be a superior source of overall health, leading to a magnetic inner glow.

Sunflower seeds are high in vitamin E, with 90 percent of the recommended daily allowance of this vitamin in a quarter cup. Vitamin E rids the body of free radicals that cause cellular damage. Vitamin E also imparts anti-inflammatory properties to sunflower seeds, essential in protecting the body from a host of beauty and health issues. Sunflower seeds contain selenium, an important trace mineral that works in conjunction with the antioxidant vitamin E and promotes DNA repair. The seeds have plentiful concentrations of magnesium, which assists in over three hundred different enzyme reactions in the body. Magnesium is a building block of health, and a lack of it can contribute to constipation, which is the death of beauty.

But it doesn't stop there. These powerhouse little seeds are also packed with fiber, vitamins B_1 and B_5, and folate. They also provide a healthy dose of copper, selenium and phosphorous, which are all important minerals. Just a quarter of a cup (four tablespoons) of seeds contains at least half the daily requirement of these important nutrients. Filled with healthy beauty fat, they are also high in amino acids to build protein in the body, which is essential for the maintenance, growth and repair of tissues. In addition, sunflower seeds contain the amino acid tryptophan, which aids in the production of serotonin, an important neurotransmitter that relieves tension and anxiety, calms the brain and promotes relaxation. Happy seeds, aren't they?

BEAUTY FOOD 49: SPROUTS

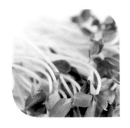

The sprouting process is the miraculous, transitional time when a seed awakens from its incubation, upon exposure to a moist, safe environment. Think of the growth of a baby for its first few months. Likewise, the sprout, which is the "baby" plant, starts to multiply its nutritive value of vitamins, minerals and amino acids, which supply abundant plant protein and many other nutrients needed to sustain the mature plant. Eating sprouts transmits these nutrients right into your body.

Sprouts are one of the most powerful foods for cellular regeneration and health. Sprouts contain an incredible range of nutrients to cleanse your body, nourish your cells and tissues, and contribute to a beautiful glow, from the inside out. Sprouts are, in essence, a predigested food whose nutrients are extremely easy for your body to assimilate and use. Concentrated, dormant proteins convert to amino acids, concentrated fats convert to fatty acids and so on. Vitamins in seeds, such as B complex and C, can be increased by up to 2,000 percent during the sprouting biochemistry that lasts several days. Sprouts supply a potent amount of antioxidants, protein, enzymes and minerals like iron, calcium and sulfur.

There are so many different sprouts out there, but my favorite is sunflower sprouts, which are sturdy, firmer and thicker in texture than other sprouts. I regularly use fenugreek, clover, alfalfa and broccoli, the last of which is said to contain as many as fifty times more of the antioxidant sulforaphane than mature broccoli by weight. That means you might get as many antioxidants in one ounce of broccoli sprouts as you would if you ate up to three pounds of fully grown broccoli(!).

I consume sprouts in some form nearly daily, and always fortify salads and recipes for my clients with sprouts. Sometimes I throw them in my Glowing Green Smoothie. You can easily buy your own seeds and grow your own in sprout bags, which is the most inexpensive way to keep a daily supply, or you can find them at any grocery store. If you purchase sprouts, wash them well.

BEAUTY FOOD 50: SPIRULINA AND CHLORELLA

Spirulina and chlorella are two algaes that compound the richly glow-producing, oxygenating and alkalizing properties found in other vegetables. They help increase cellular regeneration and create a beautiful, healthy glow.

Spirulina

Spirulina is in the family of blue-green algae, and is found in both the ocean and fresh water. It provides an abundant supply of many different phytonutrients. Because it contains no cellulose in its cell walls, its nutrients are easily assimilated into the body. Spirulina boasts around a 60 percent dry weight of protein, supplying the most concentrated source of protein known to man, without the energy-zapping effects of heavy animal proteins.

Found in a flake, tablet and powdered form, spirulina is densely packed with protein. It is a particularly rich source of iron, as well as other vitamins and minerals, including B complex, D and K. Spirulina is one of the richest sources of natural beta-carotenes, those potent antioxidants that convert to vitamin A in the body, and has around ten times the concentration that's found in carrots. Spirulina is also rich in iron, magnesium and trace minerals.

Toxins and heavy metals from the environment can weigh you down, diminishing your natural glow. Some researchers have found that spirulina possesses potent detoxifying properties and can cleanse mercury and other heavy metals and toxins out of the body. At the same time, it's extremely rich in antioxidants, fighting free radicals that can damage your cells. Because of its high level of protein and other nutrients, spirulina contributes to greater stamina and can help curb hunger. It can be especially helpful if you are an athlete, consumed in conjunction with demanding workouts.

One of the sure ways to improve your glow factor is to heighten your body's ability to cleanse while optimizing digestion. Research has shown that spirulina contributes to both cleansing and digestion by helping to suppress the overgrowth of bad bacteria like

Oxygen and Disease

Double Nobel Prize winner Dr. Otto Warburg found that the growth of cancer cells was initiated by a lack of oxygen, and discovered that these cells, as well as viruses and bacteria, couldn't live in an alkaline and oxygen-rich environment. The foods you eat are a primary way of influencing the pH environment of the body. Seeds and nuts, before sprouting, are somewhat acid-forming in the body, due to their powerful, protective enzyme inhibitors. The sprouting process allows them to become alkalizing in your body. Sprouts and other raw plant foods have a powerful alkalizing affect on your body, support cellular regeneration and bring abundant oxygen into your body.

E. coli and Candida yeast, and promoting the growth of friendly flora that optimize nutrient absorption and increase immunity.

A regimen including spirulina was found to be helpful to those working on the cleanup effort of the 1986 Chernobyl disaster who experienced overall radiation damage.[4] In 1994, a Russian patent was awarded for spirulina as a medical food to reduce allergic reactions from radiation sickness. Two hundred and seventy children from Chernobyl, consuming five grams a day for forty-five days, lowered their radionucleides by 50 percent and normalized allergic sensitivities.[5] While you may not be subject to a nuclear disaster, you do want to take extra measures to feel and look your best, since chemicals and pollutants are teeming in the food and water supply, as well as in the environment.

The gamma-linolenic acid (GLA) present in spirulina may help balance hormones, dissolve fat deposits, prevent heart problems and reduce bad cholesterol. Regular consumption of spirulina can help stimulate immunity and wound healing.

A general recommended amount is one to five grams per day, but start with small amounts to determine what works best for your body. Don't cook spirulina because that will destroy some of its nutrients. The powdered form is great to work into recipes—be sure to check out the delicious Spirulina Pie Recipe on my website, as well as Spirulina Salad Dressing and Spirulina Shots in Part III.

Chlorella

A single-celled algae, chlorella derives its name directly from its high levels of chlorophyll, making it a top detoxifying and glow-promoting food. Chlorophyll is one of the most important compounds for producing a beautiful glow. It helps carry oxygen around the body, which is important for radiance, and helps prevent the withered, unhealthy look of anemia. Chlorella is more densely packed with chlorophyll than any other plant. This is a really important compound for cleansing the digestive tract (helping to prevent constipation), as well as for promoting liver function and blood flow. Unpasteurized chlorella also contains many different types of enzymes.

Chlorella is extremely alkalizing in the body and helps combat the deleterious effects of acidic elements in the diet, including processed foods, sodas and animal products. Thus, chlorella can help balance your pH, especially if your diet is transitioning or is not in balance. At around 50 percent protein, but containing all essential amino acids to form a complete protein, chlorella is slightly lower in protein than spirulina. However, it is higher in chlorophyll, so both algaes are extremely useful in different ways. Chlorella also contains the B vitamins, vitamin E and carotenoids. Unlike spirulina, chlorella contains vitamin C. It, too, is a rich source of many minerals, including the beauty minerals magnesium, zinc and iron, which contribute to healthy skin and blood flow, to promote better circulation and a glowing complexion.

Chlorella has potent detoxifying properties, such as the ability to help eliminate heavy metals and other toxins from the body, which weigh you down, cause you to age faster and reduce your essential luster. Its fibrous material binds to heavy metals, toxins and pesticides that accumulate in your body. This keeps the digestive tract and other eliminative organ channels clean, which contributes to healthy blood and ensures that metabolic wastes are efficiently expelled from the tissues and organs. Chlorella can further be a potent aid in improving digestion, promoting healing and fighting candidiasis (see Chapter 2).

Chlorella has a wide range of many different carotenoids, far more than just beta-carotene. Many people are deficient in magnesium, and chlorella provides a rich source of this mineral, which is important for energy production and muscle strength, among other functions. Research has found that high cholesterol levels and blood sugar metabolism are helped by daily consumption of chlorella.[6] As with spirulina, chlorella helps stimulate the friendly flora in your gut and promotes a good balance of healthy bacteria in your system.

Chlorella is conveniently available in tablet form. I carry it in my purse sometimes, and when I get into a bind and am hungry, I'll eat a few to help ward off hunger. Some have associated chlorella with weight loss, due to its high level of satiating nutrients.

Recipes for Inner Glow

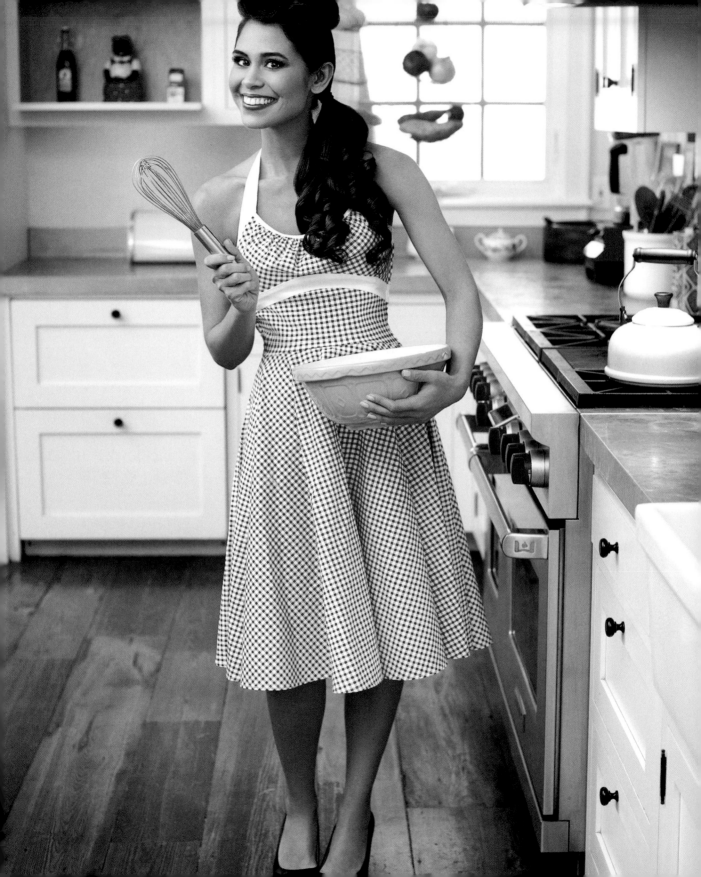

PUTTING IT ALL TOGETHER: SHOPPING AND MEAL PLANS

9

This chapter helps you get ready to put the ideas in the first two parts of this book into practice, so that you can make the recipes and have renewed energy, clearer skin, reduced under-eye circles, shinier hair and a healthy and radiant glow.

GOING SHOPPING

As you transition the way you eat, you'll find yourself shopping in a whole new way. But for now, consider stocking up on the beauty foods discussed in Part II, and also purchasing the ingredients listed in the recipes you want to make.

NOTE ON ORGANIC: Please be sure to buy as much organic as you can afford or is accessible. If budget is an issue, see page 11 for tips on which produce is the most important to buy organic. My website also has additional budget shopping tips.

BEAUTIFUL SKIN

YOUTHFUL SKIN

- [ ] Red bell peppers
- [ ] Coconut (water, whole young coconuts, oil in small amounts)
- [ ] Avocados
- [ ] Spinach

RADIANT SKIN

- [ ] Watercress
- [ ] Figs
- [ ] Sweet potatoes
- [ ] Cucumbers
- [ ] Acai

SOFT SKIN

- [ ] Pineapple
- [ ] Almonds
- [ ] Walnuts
- [ ] Flaxseeds

UNLINED, WRINKLE-FREE SKIN

- [ ] Pears
- [ ] Cabbage
- [ ] Turmeric

CLEAR, BLEMISH-FREE SKIN

- [ ] Probiotic & Enzyme Salad, Ginger and Caraway Seed Variety
  - [ ] Green or purple cabbage
  - [ ] Gingerroot
  - [ ] Caraway seeds
- [ ] Arugula

- [ ] Onions
- [ ] Raw apple cider vinegar
- [ ] Garlic
- [ ] Lemon

BEAUTIFUL HAIR

- [ ] Pumpkin seeds
- [ ] Dulse
- [ ] Carrots
- [ ] Radishes
- [ ] Nutritional yeast

BEAUTIFUL EYES

BRIGHT EYES

- [ ] Papaya
- [ ] Beets
- [ ] Blueberries
- [ ] Apples

ELIMINATING DARK CIRCLES AND PUFFINESS

- [ ] Celery
- [ ] Collard greens
- [ ] Asparagus
- [ ] Bananas

BEAUTIFUL BODY

FLUID BODY MOVEMENT

- [ ] Broccoli
- [ ] Brussels sprouts
- [ ] Sesame seeds
- [ ] Romaine lettuce

CELLULITE-FREE BODY

- [ ] Glowing Green Smoothie
  - [ ] Romaine lettuce
  - [ ] Spinach
  - [ ] Celery
  - [ ] Apples
  - [ ] Pears
  - [ ] Bananas
  - [ ] Lemon
- [ ] Fresh cilantro
- [ ] Fresh parsley
- [ ] Buckwheat
- [ ] Oat groats (or steel-cut oats)

TONED BODY

- [ ] Kale
- [ ] Hemp seeds
- [ ] Quinoa
- [ ] Millet
- [ ] Chia seeds

INNER GLOW

- [ ] Bee pollen
- [ ] Sunflower seeds
- [ ] Sprouts
- [ ] Spirulina
- [ ] Chlorella

PREPARING YOUR KITCHEN

You won't necessarily need many new kitchen appliances to get started, but there are a few essentials whose benefits will come back to you a hundredfold. When you have good equipment, it makes food preparation easier and helps make your food taste better, so you are more inspired to stick with the program. For additional product options and more product recommendations for multiple categories, visit my website at www.kimberlysnyder.net.

BLENDER

An excellent blender is the number one most important piece of kitchen equipment you'll need. You'll be using a blender to create the Glowing Green Smoothie and other smoothies, raw soups, salad dressings, nut pâtés, and more.

My absolute favorite blender is the Vitamix. The Glowing Green Smoothie comes out silky smooth and tastes absolutely delicious using the Vitamix. It is so powerful it efficiently breaks down and allows you to derive the maximum nutritional benefit from your produce. Although it's an investment, it will last you forever and is truly invaluable. It's also really easy to clean. And here's a great tip if you are on a tight budget: you can purchase a refurbished Vitamix at a much lower cost on the company's website. It's almost the same quality as a new one and comes with the same seven-year warranty. Go to kimberlysnyder. net/blog/vitamix and you will automatically get free standard shipping.

If you are on a super tight budget and even a refurbished Vitamix is not an option, here are some lower-priced blenders in pricing order that you can check out: The KitchenAid, around $140; the Ninja, around $100; and the Magic Bullet, around $50. Please note that while all these lower-cost options have the ability to make the Glowing Green Smoothie, your results may vary from model to model.

JUICER

You'll be using a juicer to make your Glowing Green Juice. (Remember that straight fruit juices are not recommended.) There are several good juicers I recommend:

◉ **Two-speed Breville juicer:** This is a good basic centrifugal juicer that is fairly easy to clean. Because it's produced by centrifugal motion, juice made from this kind of juicer should ideally be consumed immediately to get the maximum benefits. If you do store juice for short periods, be sure to keep it cool and covered, and drink it as soon as you can.

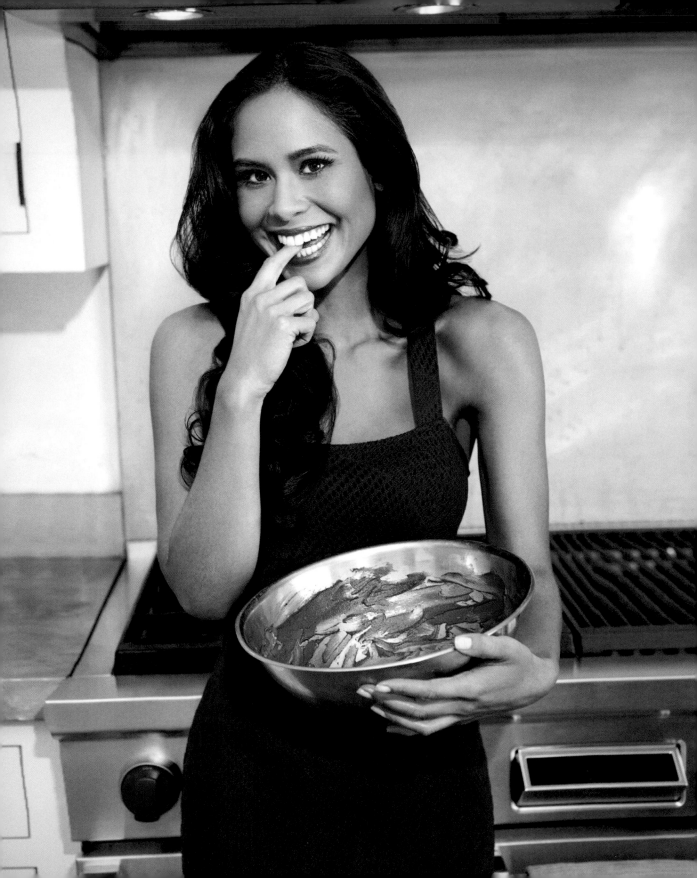

- ⊙ **Hurom slow juicer:** This juicer extracts juice by first crushing the plant matter and then squeezing the pulp to extract more juice, albeit somewhat time-consuming.

- ⊙ **Norwalk juicer:** This is a superior juicer, as it uses a hydraulic press to squeeze juice out of the plant fiber in a cold-pressed method rather than crushing the cell walls at higher heat, as other juicers do. The main advantage is that the juice oxidizes at a much slower rate, so enzymes remain intact for much longer and the juice can be stored longer. You'll also get a higher yeild of juice out of your produce. However, the cost is upwards of $2,500.

FOOD PROCESSOR

This is an important kitchen tool that serves different functions from a blender. Food processors are better for mixing ingredients (rather than fully liquefying or emulsifying them) and are ideal for preparing certain nut pâtés, bread crumbs, veggie burgers, crusts or anything that needs to retain some texture. If you're on a budget, invest your money in a blender, and then think of adding a food processor down the line. My favorite brand is Cuisinart.

SALAD SPINNER

Soggy salads are just not appetizing. This tool whips all that excess water right off lettuce and other greens so you're inspired to eat more salads. I also use the inner strainer to wash my fruits and vegetables when I make the Glowing Green Smoothie and Glowing Green Juice.

DEHYDRATOR

A dehydrator is simply a box with a fan and a small electric heater, in which food is laid on trays. It slowly "bakes" the moisture out of food over many hours at low temperatures (I usually keep mine on 105°F), preserving all the foods' natural enzymes and creating raw breads, crackers and desserts. If you're interested, the Excalibur brand is a good one. Teflex sheets are very helpful as well, so I'd advise you to purchase them along with a dehydrator. They are the washable sheets that you place the foods on and lay on the trays of the dehydrator. The other alternative to buying a dehydrator is to keep your oven on the lowest setting with the door cracked open when dehydrating food.

A FEW LAST TIPS

Here are a few additional thoughts on the recipes:

- ◎ **Sweet stuff:** You'll see that the sweetener I use for almost all my recipes is stevia, both in liquid and powdered form. I like having both forms on hand, but you can see which works better for you. Stevia can be an acquired taste, but I've found that my and my clients' taste buds really have shifted over time as we've moved away from sugar and artificial sweeteners. If you're transitioning and are having a hard time with stevia, for some reason, I would say that xylitol or erithrytol crystals, which are natural sugar alcohols, are the next best option and work well in baking. But don't give up on stevia! Over time, you may grow to love it as I do. Some brands taste far better than others.

  When a liquid sweetener is what you're looking for, my go-to product is raw coconut nectar, which is rich in minerals and amino acids, has a low impact on blood sugar levels and is also low in fructose. It is now available in most health food stores. If you have trouble finding it, you can always substitute maple syrup. However, I don't recommend agave (ever!) as a substitution, for reasons found in Chapter 2.

- ◎ **Salt:** In most recipes, I tend to encourage adding salt "to taste" rather than giving a specific amount. The reason is that your salt tolerance may start to shift. I now add very little (or no) salt to my own food; instead, I often add in chopped scallions or whole dulse leaves to add a salty flavor without too much sodium.

  I encourage you to use as little salt as possible and work to cut down if you are used to heavily salting your food. Not only will it be better for your blood pressure and heart health, but it will also help keep you from looking puffy under your eyes and throughout your body. Sodium can create "false fat" by encouraging fluid retention, making you look up to *nine pounds* heavier than you truly are. When you cut back on salt, over time you'll realize you don't need as much of it as you thought you did.

- ◎ **Tamari:** When I wrote a recipe for a popular magazine that included tamari and the editor told me she had no clue what tamari was, I figured I better mention it here.

  Tamari is a fermented soybean product, which was actually first discovered as a by-product of producing miso. The fermentation process breaks down many of the key allergy-triggering proteins in the soybeans. Tamari adds a rich flavor to recipes and is gluten-free. In contrast, regular soy sauce and nama shoyu contain wheat, and therefore gluten. Look for tamari in the Asian section of supermarkets, and always go for the low-sodium varieties.

- ⊙ **"Weird" baking ingredients:** Vegan and gluten-free baking is no easy task. Without the sticky, binding qualities of gluten and items like egg whites, a combination of other flours and ingredients are needed to create baked items.

The ingredients listed—xanthum gum, arrowroot starch, tapioca starch—may not be what you're used to baking with, but they are excellent binders and can be found in health food stores and online. A little goes a long way, so you don't have to buy them often. Ener-G egg replacer is also found in most health food stores, and is the best vegan and non-soy egg replacer I've found. With a little effort, you, too, can find these ingredients and create easily digestible, delicious baked goods.

For much more information on shopping tips and specific brands I recommend, please be sure to visit the online Resources section at www.kimberlysnyder.net.

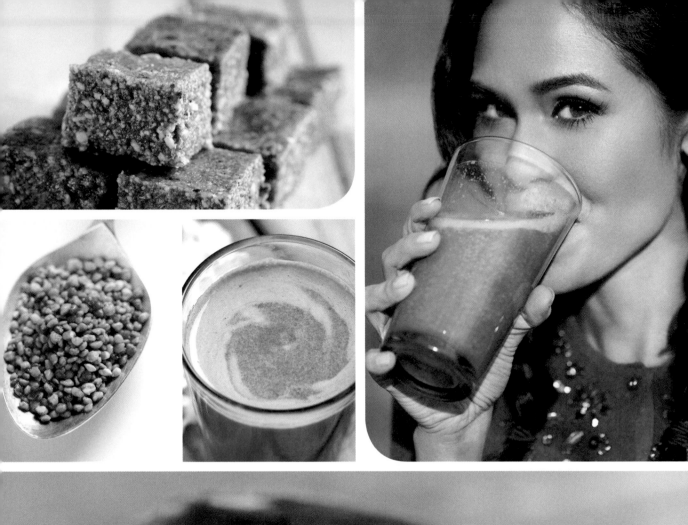
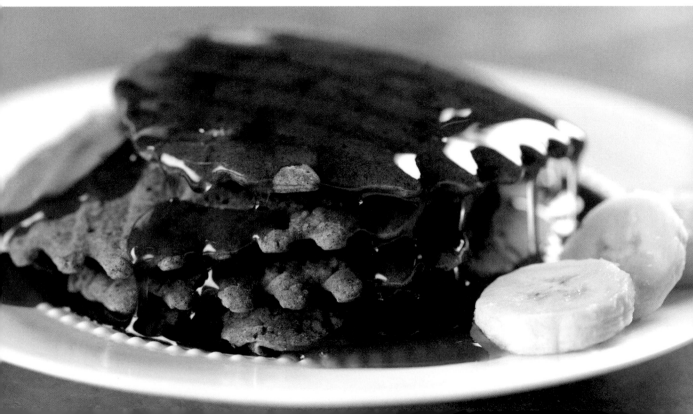

BEAUTY SMOOTHIES AND ENERGY BOOSTERS

10

GLOWING GREEN SMOOTHIE

YIELD: ABOUT 60 OUNCES

INGREDIENTS

2 cups very cold, filtered water

7 cups chopped spinach (about a medium bunch)

6 cups chopped romaine lettuce (about 1 small head)

1½ cups chopped celery (about 2 stalks)

1 apple, cored and chopped

1 pear, cored and chopped

1 banana

2 Tbs. fresh lemon juice

OPTIONAL INGREDIENTS

Ice cubes (if you prefer beverages on the colder side, but only add as few as you need)

½ cup chopped cilantro (stems okay)

½ cup chopped parsley (stems okay)

This is it . . . the star of the whole Beauty Detox program! This is the drink I have every day, and that I urge all my clients to drink daily to feel and look their best. I hope it will become part of your daily routine as well.

I generally recommend starting out consuming around 16 ounces of the Glowing Green Smoothie, and then working up to 24 ounces or more (depending on your size, appetite, metabolism and activity levels). Personally, I usually drink up to 32 ounces through the morning, and avoid other foods until lunch, except maybe some fruit. A Vitamix blender is definitely recommended to make this smoothie, so that it's smooth, silky and delicious in only a few minutes of prep time and cleanup (see Chapter 9 for more information). I just love seeing my Vitamix full of the green magic that makes my skin glow, makes my hair healthy and makes me feel like a million bucks. Sixteen ounces of Glowing Green Smoothie supplies over 13 grams of cleansing, precious fiber.

The advantages of making a big batch like this one are time and convenience. Unlike juice, which has a short nutritional life span, the Glowing Green Smoothie will keep in your refrigerator, as long as it's covered, for about two and a half days. You can share it with your family or roommates, or have it yourself over that period. You can also freeze individual portion–size containers and thaw it out the night before if you're in a bind. Make sure plastic containers are BPA-free; BPA is a chemical that can tamper with hormones.

NOTE: I encourage you to mix and match your greens and fruit. Vary this recipe with kale, chard, arugula and the like. Just avoid melons, as they are a specific type of fruit that digests better on their own.

DIRECTIONS:

⊙ Add water, chopped spinach and chopped romaine to the blender. Starting the blender on a low speed, mix until smooth. Gradually move to higher speeds and add the herbs (if using), celery, apple and pear. Add the banana and lemon juice.

NOTE: The reason I encourage blending the greens first is to ensure they have the most time to break down. The fruit is made of simple sugars and water and doesn't need to be blended as long.

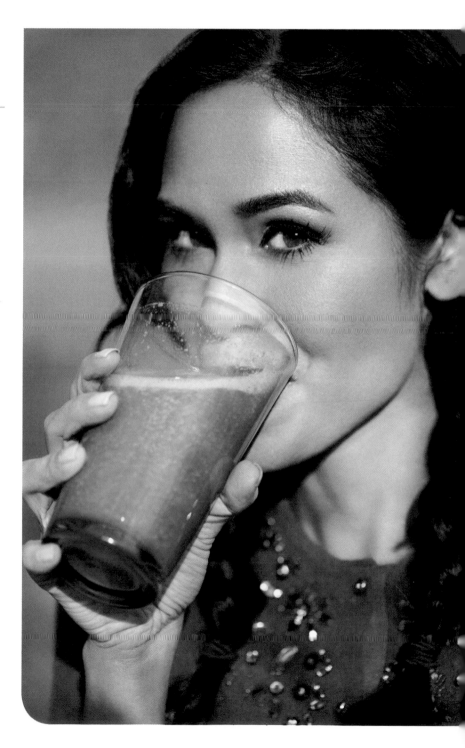

GLOWING GREEN SMOOTHIE, 1 SERVING

YIELD: ABOUT 24 OUNCES

If you don't want to make a whole pitcher and just want to make enough for yourself, try this recipe. It's delicious! Sip this throughout the morning or save some for the afternoon.

INGREDIENTS

1 cup filtered or spring water

2 cups chopped spinach

1 cup chopped romaine lettuce

½ cup chopped celery

1 small pear
(or ½ a large one)

½ banana

1 Tbs. fresh lemon juice

DIRECTIONS:

⊙ Add water, chopped spinach, chopped romaine and chopped celery to the blender. Starting the blender on a low speed, mix until smooth. Gradually move to higher speeds and add the pear, then the banana and lemon juice.

SPIRULINA SHOTS

YIELD: SIX 2-OUNCE SHOTS

I make these green shooters for some of my actors during movie shoots, especially one actor in particular. She strongly believes her regular spirulina shots help her skin and hair look their best.

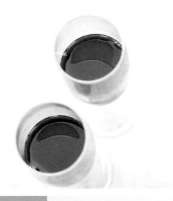

INGREDIENTS

1½ cups coconut water

1 Tbs. spirulina powder (or more, if you like)

¾ tsp. powdered or about 20 drops liquid stevia (or more), to sweeten

DIRECTIONS:

⊙ Put all ingredients in a blender and blend well. Keeps in refrigerator, covered, for a few days. Mix thoroughly before drinking.

GLOWING GREEN SMOOTHIE, LOW SUGAR

YIELD: ABOUT 60 OUNCES

This is the version of the Glowing Green Smoothie that's perfect if you're a Blossoming Beauty or suspect you may have candidiasis. Green apples, like Granny Smith apples, are sour and low in sugar. Feel free to add as much liquid stevia as you need to make your smoothie delicious.

I encourage you to mix and match your greens, as you do with the regular Glowing Green Smoothie. Whatever you do, don't add grapefruit, another low-sugar fruit. I tried that once with a client, and he told me it was absolutely horrendous. Your best bet for your one lower-in-sugar fruit choice is to stick with the green apple, unless you want to try going all green. It's the new black.

DIRECTIONS:

◉ Add the water, chopped spinach and chopped romaine to the blender. Starting the blender on a low speed, mix until smooth. Gradually move to higher speeds and add the chopped cucumber or celery, the green apple, lemon juice and stevia. Taste the smoothie, and add additional stevia if needed.

INGREDIENTS

2½ cups very cold, filtered water

9 cups chopped spinach (about 1½ medium bunches)

8 cups chopped romaine lettuce (about 1½ small heads)

2 cups chopped cucumber or celery

1 green apple, cored and chopped

2 Tbs. fresh lemon juice

Liquid stevia, to taste

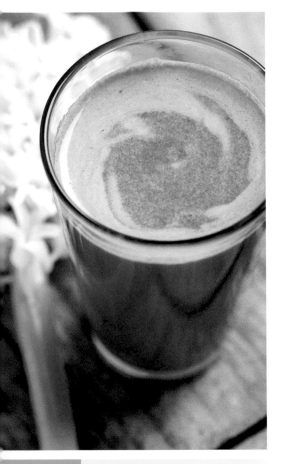

GLOWING GREEN JUICE

YIELD: ABOUT 16 OUNCES

Juicing is a different way of processing produce from blending, and the Glowing Green Juice should not be stored (as the Glowing Green Smoothie can be for a few days). Drink this juice within 15–25 minutes of making it to ensure the full preservation of its enzymes (unless you have a cold-pressed juicer). Over time, you can increase the recipe and work up to 24 ounces or more of Glowing Green Juice each day. I encourage you to mix and match your greens and produce, as you do with the Glowing Green Smoothie.

DIRECTIONS:

⊙ Run all ingredients through a juicer, putting one piece of produce at a time through the mouth of the juicer. The juice will pour into a container, which you can then pour into a glass to drink (the fiber will be dumped into another container that can then be discarded). With juice, the order in which you add the produce doesn't matter.

INGREDIENTS

8 cups chopped spinach or kale

2 cups chopped celery (about 2½ stalks) or cucumber (about ½ of one)

½ a large or 1 small lemon (cut off peel before you put it through the juicer)

1 small apple or liquid stevia, to taste

POWER PROTEIN SMOOTHIE

YIELD: ONE 24-OUNCE SERVING

I don't recommend consuming commercially processed protein powders, which are usually made with soy or whey (dairy). However, raw hemp and raw protein powders made from non-soy plant ingredients such as brown rice and sprouts are great forms of protein that are easily assimilated by your body and efficiently used. Chia seeds provide complete protein, as well as fiber, minerals and long-burning fuel (see Chapter 7 on why chia seeds are a top food for a toned body).

This drink supplies upwards of 20 grams of high-quality plant protein (depending on the type of protein powder and how much almond milk you use). It's great as a snack before working out or in the afternoon when you need something more filling during that long stretch before dinner.

Acai is a fatty fruit. Therefore, it combines well with the protein in this smoothie, as opposed to high-water fruits that contain no fat.

The addition of bee pollen and all its fantastic nutrients, enzymes and amino acids would elevate the super-charging benefits of this smoothie even more.

DIRECTIONS:

⦿ Add the almond milk and/or water to the blender first, then the other ingredients. Blend until smooth.

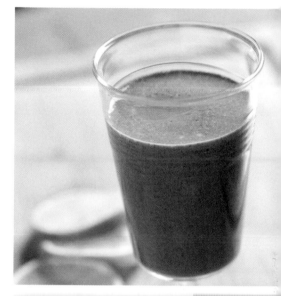

INGREDIENTS

2 cups unsweetened almond milk or water, or a 50/50 combination

3–4 Tbs. hemp or brown rice protein powder (check serving size on label)

1–2 Tbs. chia seeds (go for the higher end if you are really active)

½ frozen unsweetened acai smoothie packet (found in the freezer section of health food stores)

Liquid stevia to sweeten

½ tsp. cinnamon

½ tsp. vanilla extract

Banana (optional)

1 Tbs. bee pollen (optional)

RAW ROLLED OAT CEREAL

YIELD: 2 SERVINGS

INGREDIENTS

½ cup raw organic oat groats or steel-cut oats, soaked overnight and rinsed well

½ avocado

¼ tsp. high-quality sea salt

½ tsp. powdered stevia or about 10 drops liquid stevia (or to taste)

1–2 Tbs. cold filtered water, as needed

This recipe is simple and tasty. It is also quite filling, because the combination of the fibrous, complex carbs of the oat groats/steel-cut oats (see Chapter 7) with a raw, fibrous, mineral-rich avocado will keep you full for a while. If you prefer cooked oatmeal, that's fine as well, and you can also sweeten it with stevia. Be sure to eat celery sticks, raw spinach or other veggies before you eat the cereal.

DIRECTIONS:

⊙ Place the soaked oats in a food processor, along with the avocado, and blend. Add the sea salt and stevia.

⊙ If you like your cereal thick and chunky, don't add the water. Otherwise, try starting with 1 tablespoon to make it a bit thinner, and then try a second tablespoon, if desired.

NOTE: For variety, you can replace the oat groats with buckwheat groats, which you must also soak overnight and rinse well.

ENERGY IN A SPOON

YIELD: ONE SPOONFUL

I have this any time I feel like a boost. Sometimes I have it in the morning, after my Glowing Green Smoothie, if I have a long stretch to lunch. I find that it acts as somewhat of an appetite suppressant. Bee pollen is one of nature's most complete foods and a top food for your inner glow (see Chapter 8). Always source it from an ethical beekeeper whose bees fly over organic, or low-pollution, land. The tiny amount of coconut oil, drizzled over the top, helps it go down well and also adds fuel and a metabolism booster, as your body will process it as energy. Chew well. This is as close to taking a spoon of nature's medicine as you can get.

DIRECTIONS:

◉ Scoop the bee pollen onto a large spoon, then drizzle the coconut oil directly over the bee pollen.

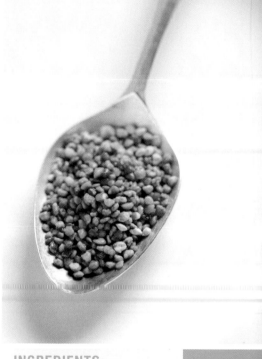

INGREDIENTS

½ Tbs. bee pollen

¼ tsp. coconut oil

GLUTEN-FREE, LOW-SUGAR SPROUTED BUCKWHEAT GRANOLA

YIELD: ABOUT 6 CUPS

INGREDIENTS

6 cups, or 32 ounces buckwheat groats

¼ cup raw coconut nectar

1 tsp. vanilla extract

3 Tbs. fresh lemon juice

1 Tbs. cinnamon

2 tsp. powdered stevia (or more, if desired)

Pinch of high-quality sea salt (optional)

NOTE: Sprouting is an important—but fairly easy—way to ensure that you're getting the full nutrition out of the buckwheat, while making it more alkaline-forming and easier to digest. It's not labor intensive at all—it really just involves filling containers with water and rinsing periodically. Not so bad, right?

Most store-bought granolas (even raw varieties) are full of copious amounts of sugar or are high in fructose, in the form of agave. The sprouting process will exponentially increase the buckwheat's enzymes and bioavailable vitamins, and will make them more alkaline and much more easily digestible. When the buckwheat starts to grow sprouting "tails," it makes me squeal with delight for having grown something on my kitchen counter (can you imagine if I were a farmer?).

I make this granola for many of my clients for press tours, as travel food, and to keep in set trailers to snack on.

DIRECTIONS:

⦿ Soak the buckwheat groats overnight in plenty of water in a large bowl on your kitchen counter. Remember that the buckwheat will absorb water, so fill the bowl with at least four inches of water above the level of buckwheat groats. Cover with paper towels or a cheesecloth to keep dust out.

⦿ The next day, rinse the buckwheat well, three times. You can use sprout bags or a strainer over a bowl for sprouting; I usually use a strainer. For six cups' worth of buckwheat, fill one large strainer or two smaller strainers, placed over bowls, so the edges of the strainers prevent the buckwheat from coming into contact with the liquid that will drip out and into the bowls. Cover with paper towels or a cheesecloth to keep dust out. If you're using sprout bags, hang them from a cabinet so they are suspended and the liquid drips down into the bowls. Every 4–6 hours (depending on the temperature and humidity of your home), place the strainers or sprout bags back in the sink and rinse the buckwheat groats thoroughly, to keep them moist. Continue this for about 24 hours (do your last rinse before you go to bed).

⊙ At the end of this 48-hour process, move your soaked and sproated groats into a large bowl. Rinse one last time. Blend or mix the rest of the ingredients until evenly distributed, and then pour over the buckwheat. Mix very well.

⊙ If you have a dehydrator, place this mixture on Teflex dehydrator sheets, and dehydrate at 105°F for 12 hours, and then stir a bit and dehydrate for another 6 hours, or until dried to the consistency you like. If you don't have a dehydrator, spread the buckwheat on a baking sheet and bake in the oven on the lowest temperature, with the door cracked open, for about 3–5 hours or more, or until dried through. Store in closed containers in the fridge. Enjoy plain or with almond or hemp milk.

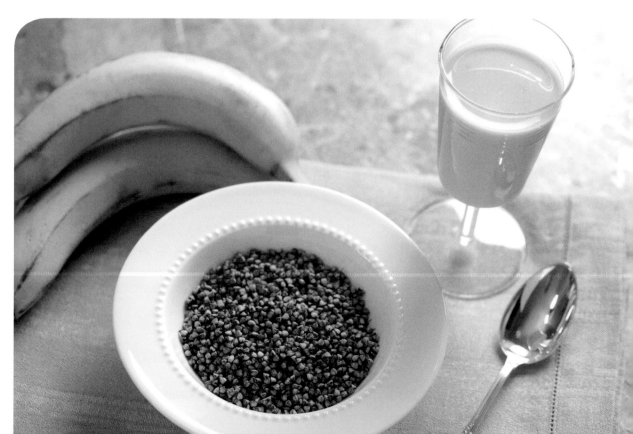

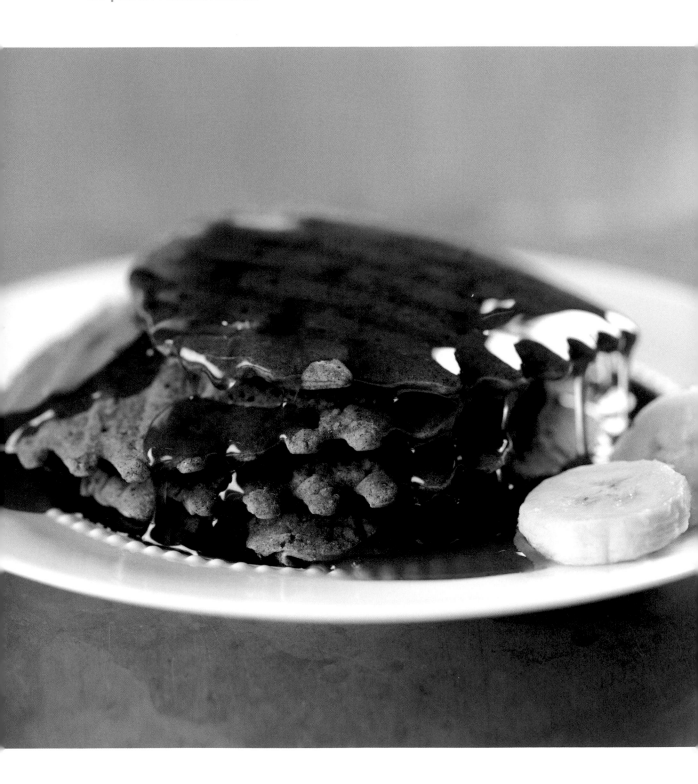

BUCKWHEAT GLUTEN-FREE VEGAN PANCAKES

YIELD: ABOUT 8 PANCAKES

Sometimes, when I'm procrastinating about writing blog posts, I wander into the kitchen and make these pancakes. They are my favorite procrastination food. They are also great if you're looking for a healthy brunch option or are just into pancakes any time of the day, the way I am.

If you need a reminder about some of these "weird" ingredients, refer back to the tips section on page 165.

DIRECTIONS:

⊙ Sift together the buckwheat flour, brown rice flour, stevia, baking powder, arrowroot starch and tapioca starch.

⊙ In a separate bowl, combine the almond milk, coconut nectar and egg replacer/water mixture. Add to the dry ingredients and whisk together until the batter is smooth. Be sure there are no lumps.

⊙ Heat a large pancake pan (or the best pan that works for you to make pancakes) to medium-high heat, and add enough coconut oil to lightly coat the bottom of the pan. Ladle out in the pan enough batter for a few pancakes and cook for 3–4 minutes before flipping the pancakes over. Cook another 2–3 minutes. Enjoy plain or topped with a bit of coconut nectar.

INGREDIENTS

1 cup buckwheat flour

½ cup brown rice flour

1½ Tbs. powdered stevia

1½ tsp. baking powder

1 Tbs. arrowroot starch

1½ Tbs. tapioca starch

1½ cups unsweetened almond milk

1 Tbs. raw coconut nectar and more for topping (optional; omit for Blossoming Beauties or if you have a hard time finding it; add a little more stevia instead)

1 Tbs. Ener-G egg replacer, mixed with 4 Tbs. very hot water

Coconut oil for cooking

ENDURANCE PROTEIN BARS

YIELD: ABOUT TWELVE 3-INCH BARS

I give these yummy bars to my actor clients when they have physically demanding roles, or when they are working out a lot and would like a sweet treat. If you are an athlete or highly active, these are a great source of energy. They are a delicious dessert or treat that can be enjoyed in moderation by non-athletes too, except for Blossoming Beauties (sorry!).

INGREDIENTS

1½ cups almonds

2 cups pecans

¾ tsp. salt

1 tsp. cinnamon

½ tsp. nutmeg

1 tsp. vanilla extract

2 dried figs, destemmed

2 dates, pitted

⅔ cup raw coconut nectar (use maple syrup instead if you can't find this)

DIRECTIONS:

◉ Preprep: Soak almonds overnight in water, then rinse well.

◉ Pulse the nuts in a food processor and process just until they are slightly chunky. Be careful not to overprocess or you'll end up with nut butter.

◉ Add the spices and vanilla extract, then the figs, dates and coconut nectar, and process until the mixture becomes evenly mixed and moist.

◉ Pour the mixture into an 8 x 8 inch glass baking dish and press in with the back of a spoon or with slightly moist hands to compress.

◉ Dehydrate at 105°F overnight for about 18 hours to harden or, if you don't have a dehydrator, place in the oven at the lowest setting, with the door cracked open a bit for about 5–6 hours, or until it hardens enough to be cut into slightly firm bars. Sometimes, if I'm in a time bind, I don't dehydrate or dry the bars at all, I just store them in the fridge and serve slightly more moist bars, which are perfectly fine to consume.

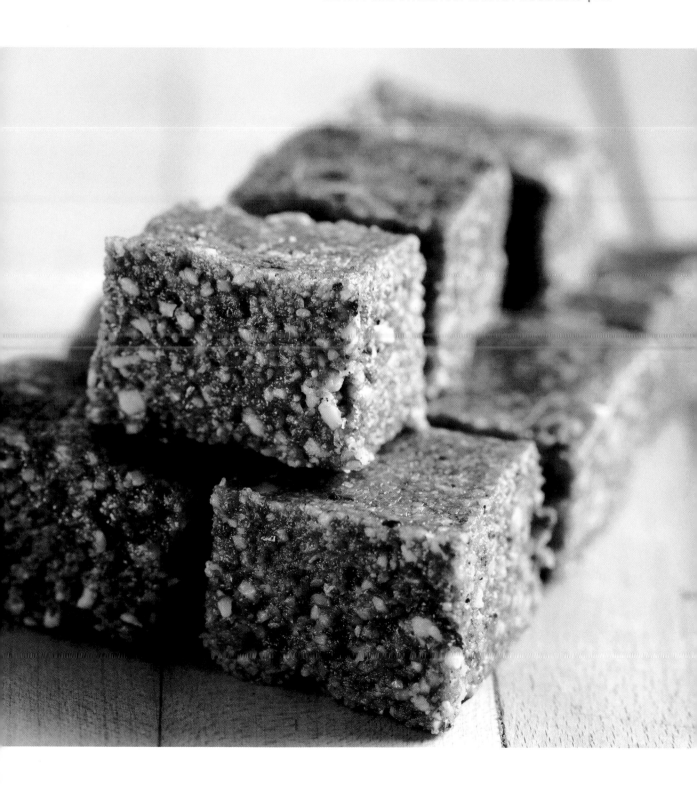

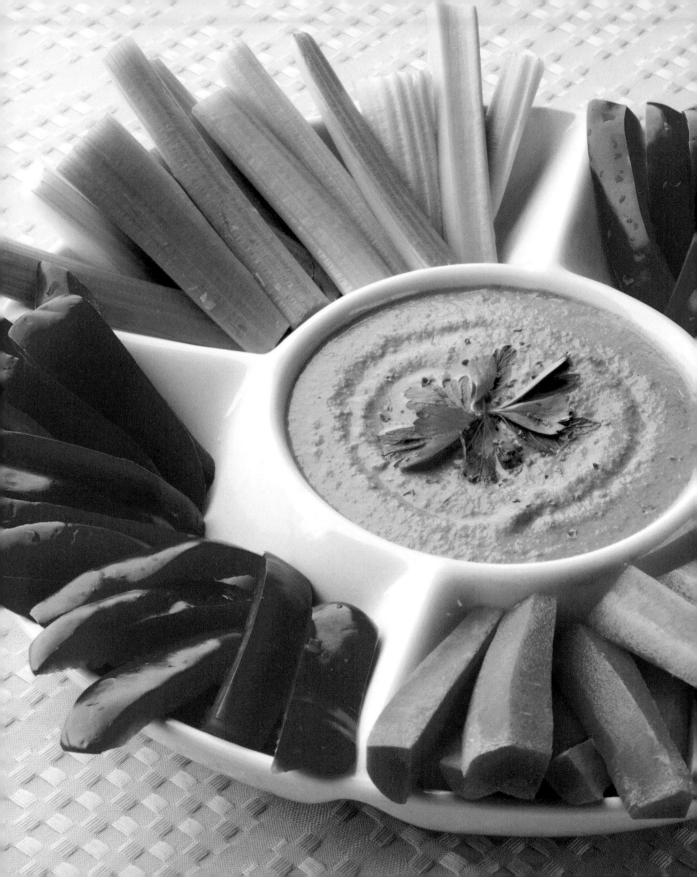

BEAUTY DRESSINGS, DIPS AND SAUCES

11

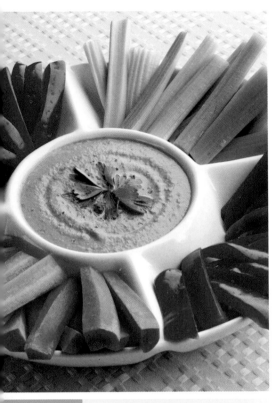

RAW MUHAMMARA DIP

YIELD: ABOUT 2½–3½ CUPS

(more or less, depending on the size of the red peppers)

This is my take on a traditional Middle Eastern dip. I think it is delicious and many of my clients agree. I keep this stocked in my fridge all the time, and I use it as a dressing and a dip. I practically drink it! Traditionally the red peppers are roasted, but because of the amazingly high content of vitamin C in red pepper, I wanted to conserve that and the rest of their nutrient content. The walnuts are usually toasted, but I'm sure it doesn't surprise you that I'd rather keep them raw, too, for our recipe. This way, you're getting the full boat of amino acids, omega fats and vitamins, completely unadulterated.

DIRECTIONS:

⊙ Combine all ingredients in a blender and blend until smooth. Adjust seasoning, as desired, and serve with raw veggies, such as celery, cucumber and carrot sticks.

INGREDIENTS

3 red peppers

1 cup raw walnuts, soaked for 15 minutes

1 medium garlic clove, peeled and minced

2 Tbs. nutritional yeast

¾ tsp. high-quality sea salt

1 Tbs. fresh lemon juice

½ tsp. powdered stevia

⅛ tsp. cayenne pepper

½ tsp. cumin

HOMEMADE BELLA MARINARA

YIELD: ABOUT 8 CUPS

This is a delicious, simple, homemade marinara sauce. You can always buy a glass-bottled variety, but I love making my own sauce when I have time.

Because you're using a small amount of olive oil, a monounsaturated fat, to cook with, be sure to use low-medium heat to sauté the onions and garlic.

To make sauces and other recipes, it's important to use fresh tomatoes and tomato paste from glass jars, avoiding canned tomatoes altogether. Bisphenol A (BPA), a synthetic estrogen associated with health issues such as reproductive complications and heart disease, is often contained in the linings of tin cans, and can leach into the tomatoes themselves. Test results from an Environmental Working Group survey detected BPA in 41 percent of canned vegetables.[1]

It's a great idea to make this first, and then while it's simmering you can make other components of your meal. Don't rush the sauce!

DIRECTIONS:

⊙ Heat oil in a large saucepan over medium-low heat. Sauté onion gently for a few minutes, until it becomes translucent. Add the garlic and sauté for about one more minute.

⊙ Add the puréed tomatoes and the tomato paste. Increase the heat until the sauce is just under a boil, and then immediately reduce heat to a simmer. Add basil, oregano, sea salt and black pepper, to taste.

⊙ Cook over low heat for 30 minutes, until the sauce has reduced and flavors are condensed.

INGREDIENTS

1½ Tbs. first cold-pressed olive oil, stored in a dark bottle

⅓ cup finely chopped white onion

2 garlic cloves, peeled and minced

14 Roma tomatoes, puréed in a blender or food processor

⅔ cup tomato paste, from a glass container

⅓ cup coarsely chopped fresh basil leaves

¼ tsp. dried oregano or 1 Tbs. fresh oregano, peeled from the stem and chopped

High-quality sea salt, to taste

Freshly ground black pepper, to taste

VEGAN CREAM CHEESE

YIELD: 1 CUP

This is a pretty awesome dairy-free, soy-free spread for those looking for a creamy replacement. It has really helped me transition some bagel and cream cheese–loving clients off their old fix. I spread it over gluten-free or raw crackers, or you can slather it on veggie sticks or use it as a base spread for a collard green and veggie wrap. Delicous!

INGREDIENTS

- 1¼ cups pine nuts
- 1 Tbs. coconut oil
- ½ tsp. sea salt
- 1 Tbs. lemon juice
- 1 very small clove garlic
- 1 Tbs. minced white onion
- 2 Tbs. water

DIRECTIONS:

⊙ Blend all ingredients together until smooth. Place in a container in the freezer for 2 hours to help set the coconut oil and achieve the right texture. After 2 hours, move to the refrigerator. Will keep about 5 days.

OIL-FREE GARLIC, RAW APPLE CIDER VINEGAR, TAHINI AND ALMOND BUTTER DRESSING

YIELD: ABOUT 1½ CUPS

Here's a dressing to get your raw apple cider vinegar on. It's creamy from the beneficial sesame seeds (what tahini is made from) and almond butter—so absolutely no need for oil.

INGREDIENTS

- 2 cloves garlic
- 1 Tbs. tamari
- 3 Tbs. raw apple cider vinegar
- ¼ tsp. high-quality sea salt
- ½ cup water
- 2 Tbs. nutritional yeast
- ⅓ cup tahini (preferably raw)
- 2 Tbs. almond butter (preferably raw or unroasted)

DIRECTIONS:

⊙ Put all the ingredients, except for the tahini and almond butter, in a blender and blend until smooth. Add the tahini and almond butter, and blend again until the dressing is thoroughly combined.

MAGENTA GODDESS DRESSING

YIELD: ABOUT 1¾ CUPS

This dressing is a brilliant, gorgeous, purple-pink color. Thanks to the inclusion of almond butter, it supplies a good boost of energizing beauty protein. As you read in Chapter 6, beets are a delectable Beauty Food that will not only help make your eyes sparkle, but also I find them to be especially supportive of female energy. Eat more beets, as in this recipe, to bring out your inner goddess.

DIRECTIONS:

⊙ Place all the ingredients, except the almond butter, in a blender and blend until smooth. Add the almond butter and blend again until thoroughly combined.

INGREDIENTS

⅔ cup water

1 very small clove garlic

2 Tbs. fresh lemon juice

½ tsp. high-quality sea salt

1 tsp. low sodium tamari

½ tsp. powdered stevia

¾ cup chopped raw beets

⅓ cup almond butter (preferably raw or unroasted)

SPIRULINA SALAD DRESSING

YIELD: ABOUT 1 CUP

Looking for a way to fit in your inner-glow sea algae spirulina? Check out this dressing. Admittedly, it may be an acquired taste, but I find that it works beautifully on mixed greens. The vitamin C in the lemon helps your body absorb the iron in the spirulina. This dressing will keep covered in the fridge for up to 2 days.

DIRECTIONS:

⊙ Put all the ingredients into a blender and blend until smooth.

INGREDIENTS

¾ cup cold, filtered water

½ tsp. high-quality sea salt

¼ tsp. xanthum gum

½ tsp. powdered stevia

2 Tbs. lemon juice

¾ tsp. spirulina powder

KIM'S CLASSIC DRESSING

YIELD: 1–2 SERVINGS

This is my favorite, go-to dressing. It is oil- and salt-free. I started adding scallions and dulse to this dressing instead of using salt or a salty condiment, and I find they add a lot of low-sodium flavor. You can vary the amounts, depending on the type of greens you are using and how big a salad you are making. Experiment for yourself with the ingredients, adjusting the quantity and the ingredients themselves to your individual preference.

INGREDIENTS

Fresh lemon juice (try starting with 1–2 Tbs.)

Nutritional yeast (I usually start with 2–3 Tbs.)

Cayenne pepper, to taste

Handful of fresh, chopped basil or dill

½ cup or more chopped green onion (both white parts and green parts)

Handful of whole dulse leaves (optional)

DIRECTIONS:

⊙ Throw all the ingredients on freshly washed salad greens and toss together well. Taste and adjust seasonings, if necessary.

CARROT-SESAME DRESSING

YIELD: ABOUT 1¼ CUPS

This makes a delicious orange-colored dressing that is a great way to get your high-calcium sesame seeds, as well as your skin and hair-beautifying vitamin A (beta-carotene) from carrots.

INGREDIENTS

1 very small clove garlic, minced

1 cup chopped carrot

3 Tbs. fresh lime juice

½ cup cold, filtered water

½ tsp. high-quality sea salt

1 Tbs. sesame seeds (ideally soaked 8 hours then rinsed)

DIRECTIONS:

⊙ Put all the ingredients into a blender and blend, adding the sesame seeds last. Blend until smooth. Enjoy!

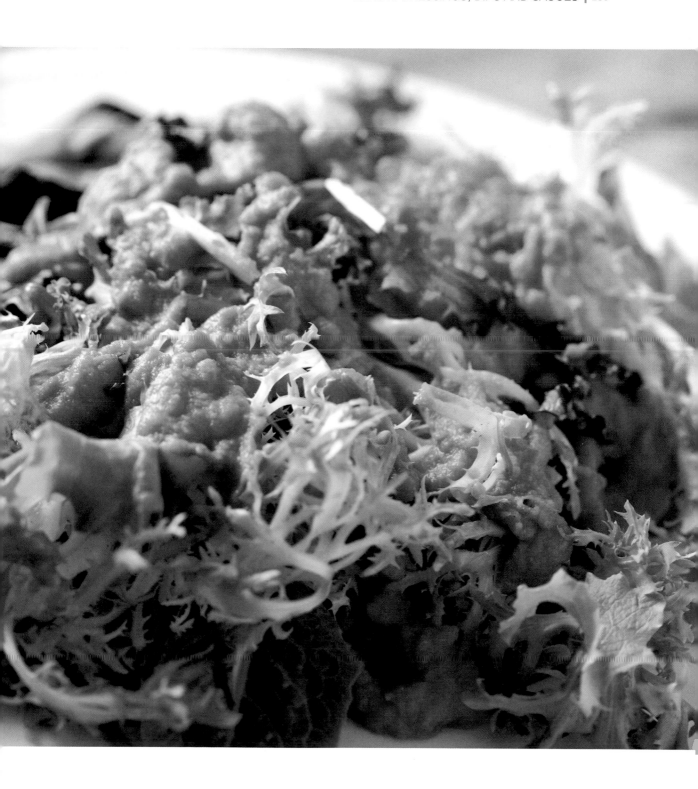

RAW, LIGHTER PESTO DRESSING

YIELD: ABOUT 1 CUP

I love the taste of pesto, but I do not love the Parmesan cheese and super-heavy douse of olive oil that usually accompanies it. This lighter version keeps its core elements, including the pine nuts, in their raw rather than cooked or roasted form, and still retains the dressing's delicious flavor.

INGREDIENTS

2 cups packed basil

3 Tbs. olive oil

2 small cloves garlic, minced

1 Tbs. nutritional yeast

⅔ cup raw pine nuts

High-quality sea salt, to taste

DIRECTIONS:

⊙ Put all the ingredients in a blender and blend to make a coarse paste—be careful not to overprocess. Enjoy over a salad or Raw Zucchini Pesto Pasta (recipe on page 288).

CREAMY DIJON-TAHINI DRESSING

YIELD: ABOUT 2¼ CUPS

Most creamy vegan dressings have a base of cashews, but I don't recommend eating cashews regularly because they are a heavy food that is often moldy and rarely (if ever) a truly raw nut. You won't even miss them in this dressing, however. Tahini is ground sesame seeds, and sesame seeds are a beauty food for moving fluidly and gracefully (see Chapter 7) and are chock full of protein and minerals. This is my and my clients' favorite creamy dressing.

INGREDIENTS

2½ Tbs. low-sodium tamari

2 Tbs. raw apple cider vinegar

1 clove garlic, minced

⅓ cup chopped white onion

⅓ cup raw tahini

¼ tsp. freshly ground black pepper

½ cup Dijon mustard

¼ cup nutritional yeast

⅔ cup water

DIRECTIONS:

⊙ Put all the ingredients into a blender and blend until smooth.

ASIAN TANG DRESSING

YIELD: ABOUT 1 CUP

This tastes just like it sounds: tangy with an Asian flair.

DIRECTIONS:

⊙ Put all the ingredients into a blender and blend until smooth.

INGREDIENTS

1 Tbs. low-sodium tamari

¼ cup unpasteurized, low-sodium miso paste

⅓ cup cold, filtered water

2 Tbs. raw apple cider vinegar

2 Tbs. fresh lime juice

1 tsp. powdered stevia or about 15–20 drops liquid stevia

¼ tsp. xanthan gum

¼ tsp. red pepper flakes

¾ Tbs. ginger, peeled and grated

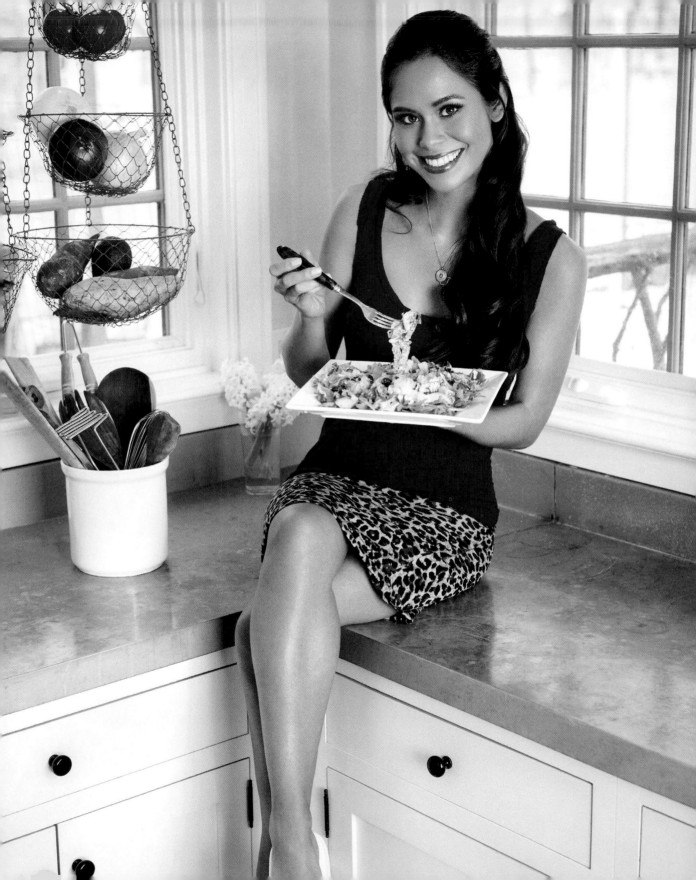

BEAUTY SALADS AND VEGGIE DISHES

12

FRESH ASIAN CUCUMBER SPRING ROLLS

YIELD: 6–8 ROLLS

INGREDIENTS

- ⅓ cup almond butter
- ½ Tbs. grated ginger
- 2 Tbs. lemon juice
- ½ tsp. + ¼ tsp. high-quality sea salt, divided
- 2 Tbs. raw coconut nectar or maple syrup
- ¼ cup raw macadamia nuts, pulsed in a food processor (Retain some texture and do not overprocess into a fine powder. Pine nuts or cashews are okay as a backup option if you can't source macadamia nuts.)
- ¾ Tbs. sesame oil
- 2 organic cucumbers, English hothouse or long garden varieties
- A few handfuls of clover sprouts
- 1 cup julienned carrots

I love the fresh rolls they make at a Thai restaurant near my apartment in New York City, which are made with rice paper and rice noodles. They certainly aren't the worst thing in the world. But when I started making my own, I wanted to use the Beauty Food cucumber, which is a potent food for brightening dull skin (see Chapter 4). I also wanted to incorporate gingery, slightly tangy and sweet flavors that I love so much in Asian food. Instead of noodles, the maca-damia nuts provide a satisfying crunch, as do the carrots and the sprouts. This is a delicious, beautiful appetizer for a dinner, or to have for lunch or a snack.

DIRECTIONS:

⊙ Put the almond butter, ginger, lemon juice, ½ tsp. sea salt and coconut nectar or maple syrup in a blender and process until smooth. Pour contents of the blender in a bowl and set aside. If you don't have a great blender, you can easily whisk the ingredients together.

⊙ Pulse the macadamia nuts in a food processor and add to a small bowl. Mix in the sesame oil and remaining sea salt, and set aside.

⊙ With a mandolin, slice the cucumbers into very thin, long strips. If you have a steady hand, you can try doing it by hand with your knife, but it is rather difficult to keep them thin and as long as the cucumber.

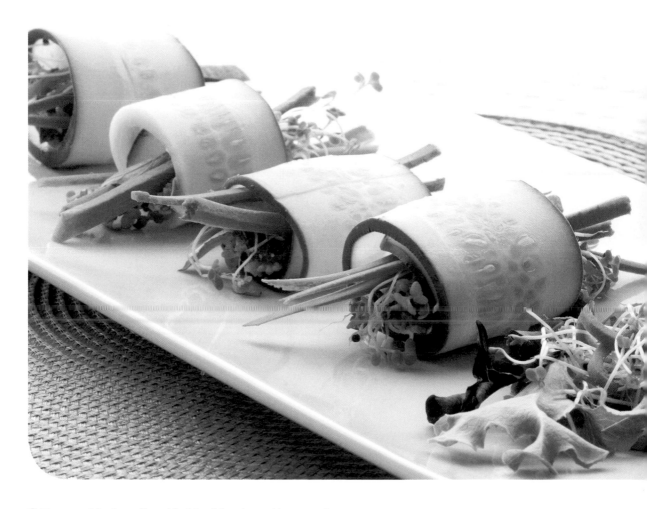

⊙ To assemble the rolls, add a bit of the almond butter mixture about one-third of the way up the cucumber slice, and top with a little bit of the macadamia nut mixture. Next, add a trace of sprouts and carrots, and roll carefully all the way up. Place on a tray with the folded edge firmly down. You may have to slightly break the outer part of the cucumber so that the roll doesn't unravel.

NOTE: If you are slicing the cucumbers by hand and they are not super-thin, it can be helpful to soak them in about 3 Tbs. of lemon juice overnight, to help soften them up for rolling.

EARTHY OREGANO KALE SALAD

YIELD: 2–4 SERVINGS

I could not love kale more than I do. I would swim in kale if I could find a big enough salad spinner.

Dharma's Kale Salad from *The Beauty Detox Solution* is one of my favorite and regular dishes, but I have branched out with this kale salad version, which is a bit more earthy-tasting and light, since it doesn't have any nutritional yeast. Do give this one a try—I think you'll like the use of oregano.

INGREDIENTS

6–8 cups lacinato kale, or 1 medium bunch of curly kale

High-quality sea salt, to taste

2 Tbs. fresh lemon juice

¾ Tbs. chopped fresh oregano

⅓ cup hemp or chopped sunflower seeds

1–2 handfuls clover, alfalfa or sunflower sprouts

1 cup cherry tomatoes, cut in half or Roma tomatoes, diced

Splash of olive oil (optional)

DIRECTIONS:

⦿ Peel the leafy part off each kale stem, and add to a large bowl. Add a pinch of sea salt to the kale and break down with your hands, tearing into bite-sized pieces.

⦿ Whisk the lemon juice, salt and oregano together in a small bowl, add the hemp seeds and mix well. Pour the mixture over the kale, add the sprouts and tomatoes, and mix well. Add a small amount of olive oil and/or sea salt, if desired, and mix well again.

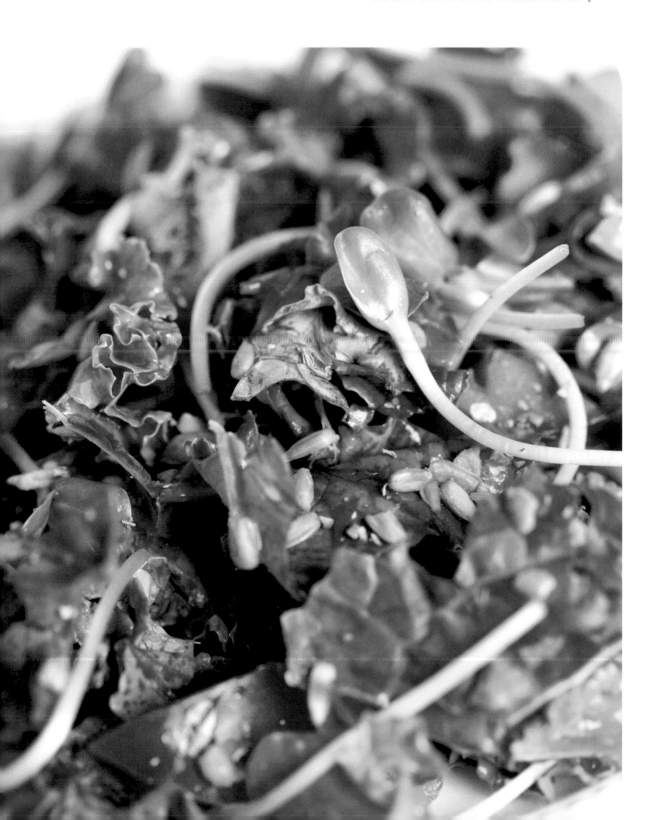

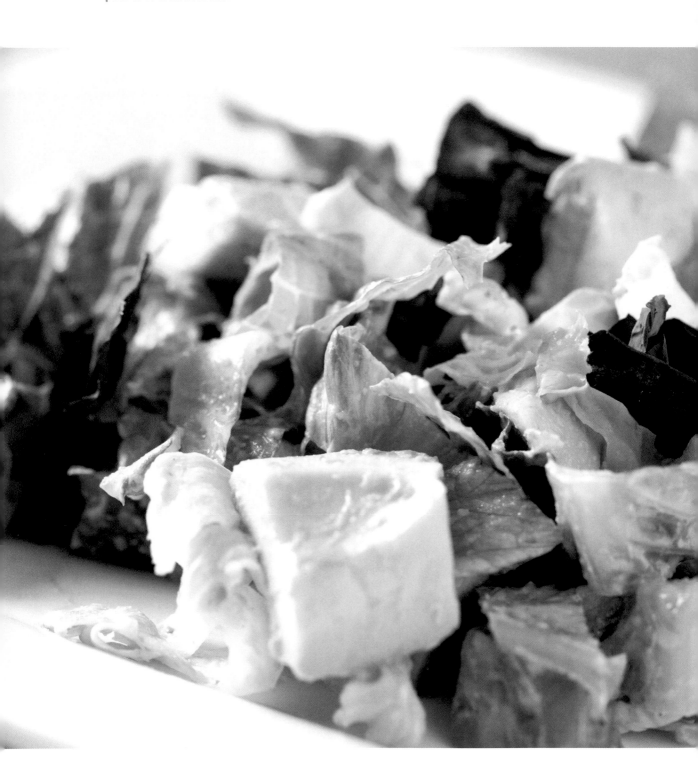

RAW VEGAN CAESAR SALAD

YIELD: 2 SERVINGS

Over the past few years, I am thrilled to report, my beloved dad has given up over 90 percent of his meat and dairy intake. He now looks about twenty years younger, and he has lost more than twenty pounds. He always loved Caesar salad, so this one's for him.

I have to add that this is a really delicious salad that many of my clients love, including some who act like eating salad is the same as pulling teeth. This salad, thankfully, is not "painful" for them.

DIRECTIONS:

⊙ Blend the dressing ingredients together until smooth. Mix the romaine hearts in a bowl with the Caesar dressing until the romaine is completely coated. Because the dressing is a thick paste, it helps to do this with clean hands to evenly cover the salad.

⊙ Add the avocado and mix well again. Top with dulse leaves.

INGREDIENTS

2 heads romaine hearts, chopped

1 medium avocado, peeled and diced

Handful whole dulse leaves, torn into small pieces (optional)

DRESSING INGREDIENTS

YIELD: ½ CUP

½ cup pine nuts

1 Tbs. miso paste

2 Tbs. nutritional yeast flakes

2 cloves garlic

¼ cup coconut water

3 drops liquid stevia

RAW PURPLE CABBAGE SLAW

YIELD: 3 CUPS

INGREDIENTS

3 cups purple cabbage, shredded

2 Tbs. apple cider vinegar

1 tsp. low-sodium tamari

1½ Tbs. nutritional yeast

3–4 drops liquid stevia

1 Tbs. tahini

OPTIONAL INGREDIENTS

½ cup finely chopped fresh parsley

¼ cup chopped pitted black olives or capers

Sliced avocado

I was never a huge coleslaw fan, as I used to think the texture was revoltingly slimy. But this version, which incorporates a light, beautifying dressing, and is made with fresh, raw purple cabbage that's practically bursting with skin-beautifying vitamin C and other nutrients, stays crispy and is appetizing and delicious. I usually eat most of it right after—and sometimes while—making it, though I do encourage you to let it marinate for a few hours before eating . . . if you can wait!

DIRECTIONS:

⊙ Shred the cabbage, using the shredding attachment on your food professor or a mandolin, or finely by hand, and place into a large bowl.

⊙ Whisk together the other ingredients, adding the tahini last. Pour over the cabbage and mix well.

⊙ Add the optional ingredients, if desired, and mix well again.

⊙ Allow to chill, covered in the refrigerator, for at least 2 hours before serving.

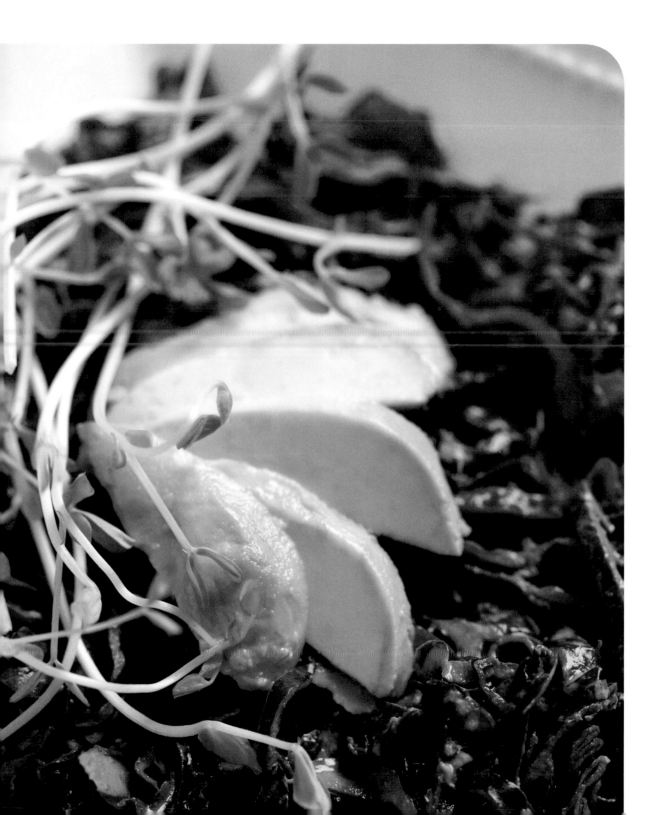

RAW BRUSSELS SPROUT SALAD

YIELD: 2–3 SERVINGS

INGREDIENTS

20 Brussels sprouts

¼ cup very thinly sliced shallots

½ cup coarsely chopped walnuts

⅔ tsp. caraway seeds

1½ Tbs. raw apple cider vinegar

1 Tbs. olive oil (optional)

High-quality sea salt, to taste

Freshly ground black pepper, to taste

I tremendously enjoy steamed and lightly roasted Brussels sprouts, but because they are so high in vitamin C, I also like to eat them raw, which most people rarely do. (Although they will still be beneficial for their mineral content, roasting will denature much of that precious vitamin C.) This is a great predinner salad, an accompaniment to something heavier, or made more substantial by adding more walnuts per serving.

DIRECTIONS:

⊙ Trim the ends from each Brussels sprout deeply, about half an inch each. Peel the leaves off individually and add to a large mixing bowl until only the inner, compactly grown leaves are left. Discard this inner part.

⊙ Add the shallots, walnuts, caraway seeds and the raw apple cider vinegar.

⊙ Add a tiny amount of olive oil, if desired, and adjust seasonings, to taste.

NOTE: This salad is best left in the refrigerator for at least 3 hours before serving, so that the raw Brussels sprouts leaves can marinate and be somewhat softened by the raw apple cider vinegar. Try to make it in the morning or early afternoon, so it can be ready by dinner.

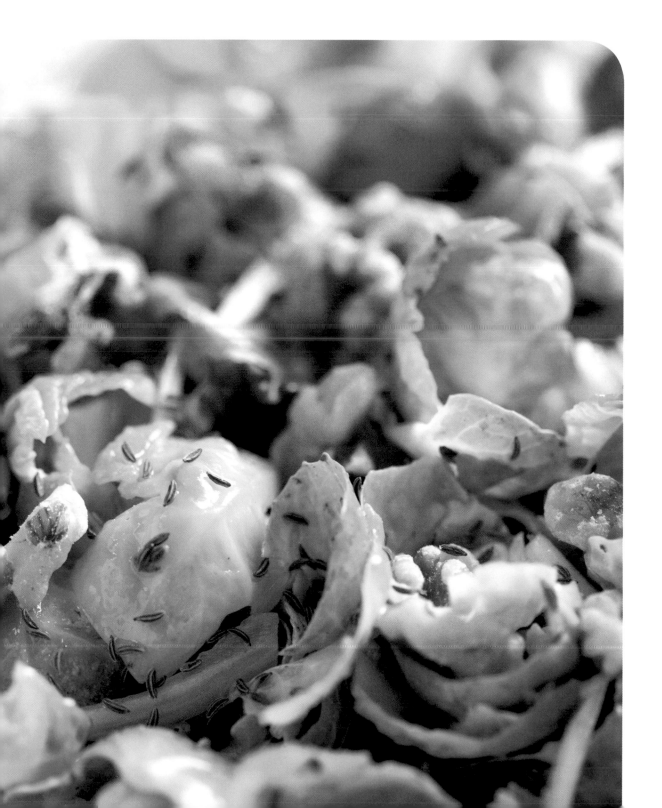

JICAMA, CUCUMBER, PAPAYA AND LIME SALAD

YIELD: 8–10 SERVINGS

INGREDIENTS

6 cups peeled and cubed jicama (about 1 medium-large jicama)

4 cups diced cucumber (peeled if not organic)

2 cups papaya, cubed

½ cup freshly squeezed lime juice

Pinch of cayenne pepper, depending on how spicy you like it

¼ tsp. powdered stevia or about 5–6 drops liquid stevia

¼ cup finely chopped fresh dill

¼ cup finely chopped fresh basil

½ tsp. lime zest, freshly grated from an organic lime

Jicama (pronounced HEE-kah-mah) is a beautifying root vegetable. It is very juicy and high in a special type of fiber called inulin, which is believed to help control blood sugar levels. Jicama also acts as a prebiotic, which is food for the friendly bacteria to balance your system. It also contains antioxidants, vitamin C, some B vitamins and small amounts of minerals, such as magnesium and iron.

For a reminder on why cucumbers are a great Beauty Food for promoting radiant skin, check out Chapter 4. Lime, similar to its citrus sister lemon, is also high in collagen-building vitamin C.

DIRECTIONS:

⊙ Mix the jicama, cucumber and papaya in a large bowl.

⊙ Whisk all the other ingredients together in a smaller bowl. Pour over the ingredients in the larger bowl and mix well. Serve over greens, as a zesty side dish or enjoy on its own.

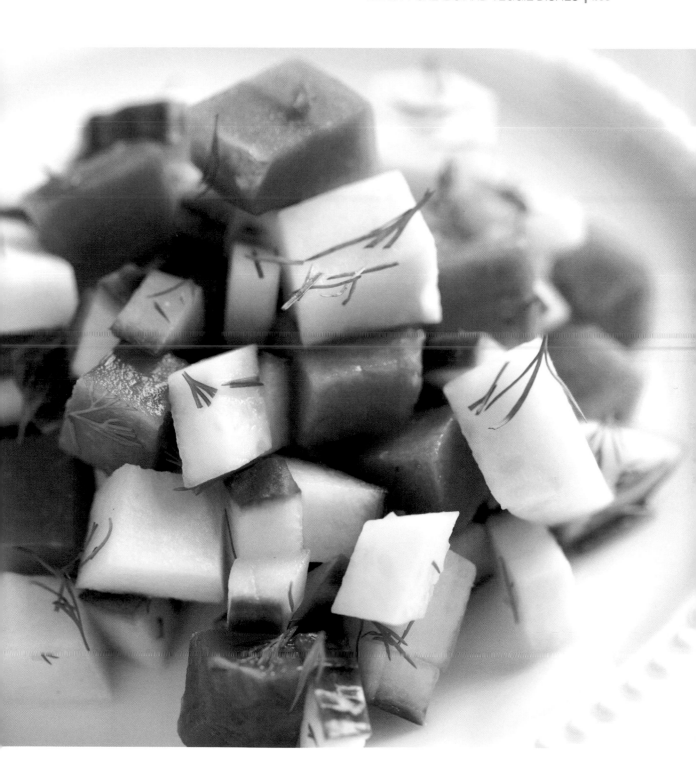

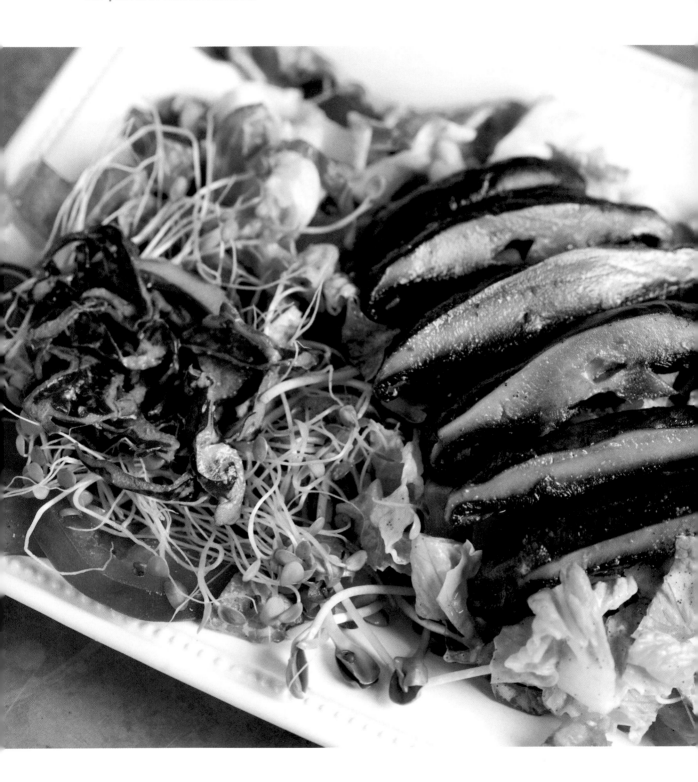

ROASTED PORTOBELLO MUSHROOM AND CREAMY DIJON-ARUGULA SALAD

YIELD: 2 SERVINGS

This is a delicious salad that's on the heartier side. I like the texture of thick slices of roasted portobello mushrooms on the salad.

DIRECTIONS:

◉ Preheat the oven to 375°F.

◉ Whisk together the cooking wine, tamari, apple cider vinegar and garlic in an 8 x 8 inch glass Pyrex or another kind of non-reactive baking pan of similar size. Marinate the mushroom caps for at least half an hour in the mixture, with the flat side down. Spoon some of the marinade over the tops, where the stem was removed, so it can really soak into the mushrooms.

◉ Take a sheet of parchment paper and lay over foil, then roll the edges so they stay together and cover the mushrooms. This prevents the foil from touching your food. Some research has shown that aluminum can leach into your food when foil is heated to high temperatures.[1] Bake for 30 minutes, keeping as much of the mixture spooned on top of the mushrooms as possible. Remove the foil and parchment paper, and bake, uncovered, for another 15 minutes. Move to a cutting board, and when the mushrooms cool down, slice into one-inch-thick pieces.

◉ Toss the arugula, tomatoes and Creamy Dijon-Tahini dressing together in a large mixing bowl, and then add the sunflower sprouts and mix again.

◉ Arrange the portobello mushroom slices neatly atop each bowl of salad. Sprinkle pumpkin seeds on top to add some crunch. Also pairs well with Raw Purple Cabbage Slaw.

INGREDIENTS

½ cup dry cooking wine

2 Tbs. low-sodium tamari

2 Tbs. raw apple cider vinegar

1 small garlic clove, minced

2 large portobello mushroom caps

Large bowl of arugula (I like to use baby arugula leaves, but you can use any greens you have on hand, like chopped romaine)

1 cup diced tomatoes

Creamy Dijon-Tahini Dressing (see page 190)

Large handful of sunflower sprouts (or another kind of sprout, if you can't find sunflower)

⅓ cup raw pumpkin seeds (ideally soaked overnight, rinsed and dehydrated or dried in the oven at the lowest temperature with the door cracked open until dried)

Handful of Raw Purple Cabbage Slaw (see page 200) (optional)

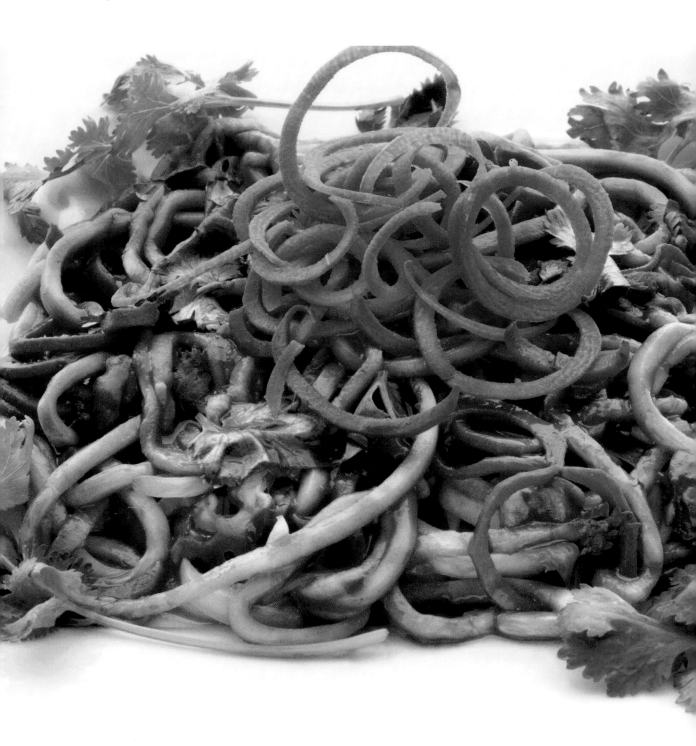

SPIRALIZED ASIAN VEGGIE SALAD

YIELD: 2–3 SERVINGS

As you can see from the picture, it appears this recipe is based on noodles. But it's not. Snap! The spiralized vegetables emulate a cold noodle dish, but this recipe cleverly replaces the noodles with beautifying veggies.

DIRECTIONS:

◉ With a spiralizer (an item you can buy for around $30 online) on the smallest chop setting, spiralize both the zucchini and the carrots and put them into a large mixing bowl. If you don't have a spiralizer, julienne the vegetables.

◉ Toss in watercress and Asian Tang Dressing. Add the walnuts and toss again. Spoon into bowls, and top each serving with a generous portion of cilantro.

INGREDIENTS

5 cups spiralized zucchini, which is about 1 large zucchini or 2–3 small zucchini

2 cups spiralized peeled carrots, which is about 3 medium carrots or 5–6 small carrots

1 cup watercress

½ cup Asian Tang Dressing (see page 191)

¾ cup walnuts, chopped

Handful of whole cilantro

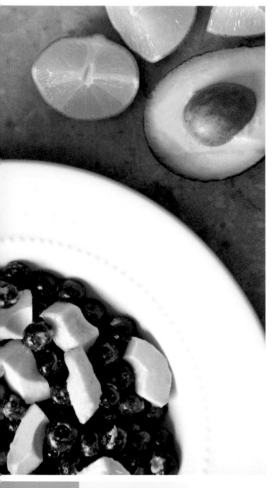

BLUEBERRY AND AVOCADO SALAD

YIELD: 2 SERVINGS

This is a very refreshing salad that I especially love to pack for the beach or picnics. I love how these two beauty fruits— and the beautifying fat in the avocado—give this salad more sustenance than a regular fruit salad.

DIRECTIONS:

⊙ Add the blueberries and avocado to a mixing bowl.

⊙ Whisk together the lime juice and stevia, and pour over the fruit. Gently toss together, being careful not to mash the avocado pieces.

INGREDIENTS

3 cups blueberries

1 medium avocado, peeled and cut into 1-inch squares

3 Tbs. fresh lime juice

½ tsp. powdered stevia or about 10–12 drops liquid stevia

KIMBERLY'S KIMCHI

YIELD: ONE 32-OUNCE MASON JAR

If you are a spice lover, this basic kimchi recipe is a good variation to alternate with the Ginger-Caraway Probiotic & Enzyme Salad for your daily allotment of probiotic-rich foods. Feel free to customize the flavors to suit your taste.

NOTE: Make sure all the jars and equipment that touch your kimchi have been sterilized at the boiling point to remove any harmful bacteria.

INGREDIENTS

3 cups coarsely chopped green cabbage

1 cup sliced carrots

½ cup chopped radishes

½ cup chopped scallions

1 jalapeño chili, seeds removed and chopped

2 inches ginger, sliced into strips

2-3 garlic cloves, chopped

½ cup cold, filtered water

3-4 outer whole cabbage leaves

DIRECTIONS:

⊙ Toss the cabbage, carrots, radishes and scallions in a large mixing bowl.

⊙ Mix the chili, ginger, garlic and water together in a small bowl and pour over the vegetables. Mix well.

⊙ Pack into the glass mason jar. Pack or pound down firmly to compress out all the air. Leave about 2 inches at the top, and fill just to that level of the compressed cabbage with cold, filtered water (do not use tap water for this because it might contain compounds that can kill the beneficial bacteria.) Fill the remaining space with the outer cabbage leaves, firmly rolled up into cylinders.

⊙ Cover the jar tightly.

⊙ Leave the kimchi in a warm cabinet, ideally around 68–70°F, for about 5 days. Remove and discard the outer cabbage leaves, and serve. The kimchi should taste tangy. Store any unused portion in the refrigerator and it will keep for at least a few weeks.

GINGER-CARAWAY PROBIOTIC & ENZYME SALAD

YIELD: ONE 32-OUNCE MASON JAR

INGREDIENTS

4 cups shredded green or purple cabbage

1 inch gingerroot, cut into strips

1 tsp. caraway seeds

Cold, filtered water

3–4 outer whole cabbage leaves

Probiotic-rich foods are one of the most important beauty foods in the whole Beauty Detox program. Get into the habit of making this salad weekly, or as often as possible, and consuming it on a daily basis. You can also buy store-bought raw sauerkraut in the refrigerated section of health food stores, but I like making my own without salt. Feel free to add a bit of sea salt, however, if that pleases your taste and motivates you to eat it more often.

NOTE: Make sure all the jars and equipment that touch your salad have been sterilized at the boiling point to remove any harmful bacteria.

DIRECTIONS:

⊙ Place the cabbage in a large mixing bowl.

⊙ Toss in the ginger and caraway seeds with the cabbage to thoroughly combine. Pack firmly into the mason jar. Every few inches, use your fist or some type of kitchen utensil to firmly press the veggies down and compress out all the air.

⊙ Leave about 2 inches at the top, and fill just to that level of the compressed cabbage with cold, filtered water (do not use tap water for this because it might contain compounds that can kill the beneficial bacteria). Fill the remaining space with the outer cabbage leaves, firmly rolled up into cylinders.

⊙ Cover the jar tightly.

⊙ Let your Probiotic & Enzyme Salad sit in a warm cabinet, ideally around 68–70°F, for about 5 days. After 5 days, remove and discard the outer cabbage leaves and serve. The salad should have a tangy taste. Store any unused portion in the refrigerator, which will keep it fresh for at least a few weeks (though if you're eating it regularly, as I recommend, hopefully your current batch should only last one or two weeks!).

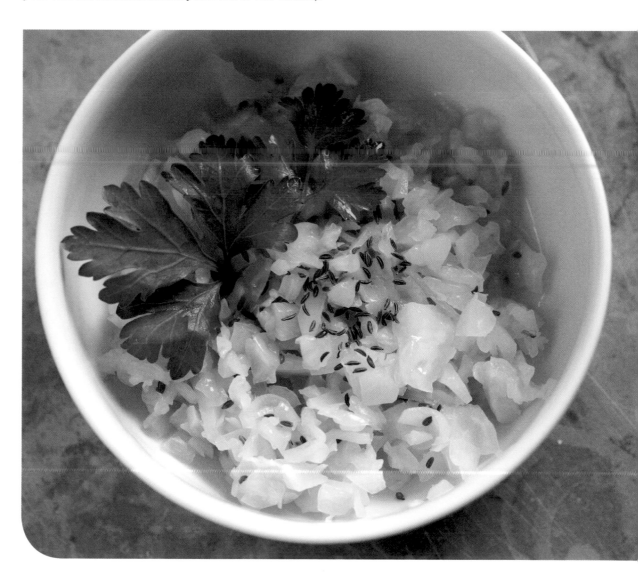

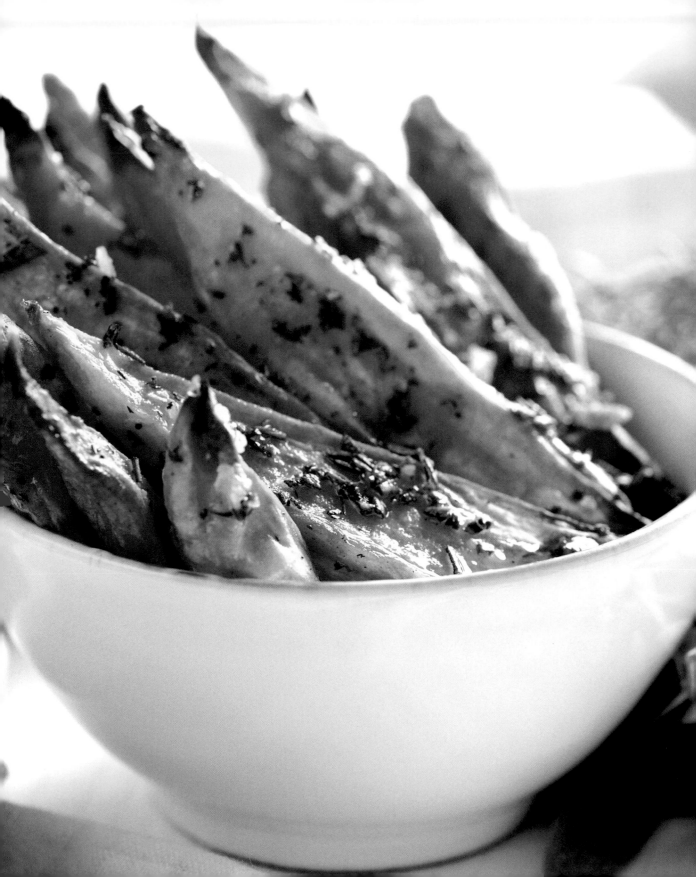

BEAUTY SIDES AND BASICS

13

GLUTEN-FREE BREAD CRUMBS

YIELD: 3 CUPS

INGREDIENTS

8–12 slices gluten-free and/or sprouted bread (for millet bread you'll need about 8 slices, while with the brown rice bread you'll need about 12 slices)

¼ tsp. garlic powder

High-quality sea salt, to taste

Pinch of dried oregano

Bread crumbs are an important component of certain recipes in the entrée section, and it is important to be able to make them in a healthy form from high-quality bread. I recommend gluten-free breads, such as millet or brown rice bread, which are typically found in the freezer section of health food markets, since they lack the heavy preservatives other breads contain. It is also a good idea to save the ends or broken pieces of these gluten-free breads in the freezer to include in your next batch of bread crumbs. I usually make them fresh when I need them for a recipe, but you could certainly store a batch in the freezer as well.

With gluten-free bread, I've found it very important to let the slices cool down completely before processing them, especially if you don't have a food processor and are making them in your Vitamix or another blender. Processing them too soon after toasting can lead to a gooey mess rather than crunchy bread crumbs.

You can choose to keep your bread crumbs plain, or add the suggested seasonings.

DIRECTIONS:

⊙ Preheat the oven to 375°F. Arrange the bread on a baking sheet. Bake for about 5–6 minutes, and then turn the slices over and bake for another 5–6 minutes to ensure they dry and bake evenly. (You may need a few minutes longer if the bread came right out of the freezer. They should brown slightly.) Remove from oven and let them cool completely, at least 30 minutes or longer.

⊙ Cut the slices into quarters, and add to the food processor. Process with the garlic powder, sea salt and oregano until you have fairly fine crumbs.

SPICY BAKED SWEET POTATO FRENCH FRIES

YIELD: 4–6 SERVINGS

During my teenage and college years, my junk food of choice was French fries. I had an elaborate rating system based on texture, crispiness and flavor that I would always relay to the amusement of my parents and friends. But now I realize that fried food not only makes you fat, it destroys your beauty.

But even knowing that, you may still love French fries. Thankfully, this baked variety made with beauty-enhancing sweet potatoes, really helps satisfy that craving. While they don't taste exactly like the deep-fried variety, the coating of arrowroot (a large perennial herb found in rain forest habitats) helps make them brown and crispy in the oven without all the deep-frying nonsense.

INGREDIENTS

2 sweet potatoes

1½ Tbs. coconut oil

1 Tbs. chili powder

½ tsp. garlic powder

Cayenne pepper, to taste

High-quality sea salt, to taste

2 tsp. arrowroot starch

DIRECTIONS:

◉ Preheat the oven to 420°F and lightly grease a baking sheet with coconut oil or use Silpat or parchment paper.

◉ Cut the sweet potatoes into thin French fries. If you make them too thick, their texture will be soggy. Try to cut them all into a uniform thickness, so that they cook evenly.

◉ In a large bowl, combine the sweet potatoes, coconut oil, chili powder, garlic powder and cayenne pepper. Use your hands to evenly coat the potatoes with the spices. Add sea salt to taste, as well as the arrowroot, and mix well again with your hands.

◉ Spread the fries out in a single layer on the baking sheet. Bake for 25 minutes, or until crispy and brown on one side. Carefully turn the fries over using a spatula, and cook for another 15–20 minutes or so, depending on how thickly you have cut them, or until all are crisp on the outside and tender inside.

MIRACLE GLUTEN-FREE VEGAN PIZZA DOUGH

YIELD: ENOUGH FOR ONE 10-INCH ROUND PIZZA

INGREDIENTS

1½ cups brown rice flour

1½ tsp. xanthan gum

1 Tbs. baking powder

½ tsp. salt

¼ tsp. powdered stevia

½ tsp. dried oregano

2 Tbs. arrowroot starch

2 Tbs. tapioca starch

¾ cup cold water

2 tsp. Ener-G egg replacer, mixed with 4 Tbs. very hot water

This pizza dough is the product of dozens of kitchen experiments, most of which ended in unfortunate results. Most gluten-free products contain high amounts of cornstarch, potato flour and egg whites as binders. When you add vegan to the mix, the eggs are out, and I don't like to use heavy amounts of corn or potato ingredients, though there is some in the small amount of egg replacer that is included.

If you're looking for the regular kind of pizza dough you are used to, you're not going to find it here. This is not like ordinary pizza dough, which is full of gluten and can easily be stretched and rolled. But what you will find is something tasty that resembles medium-thick pizza dough and will bake well.

DIRECTIONS:

⊙ Preheat the oven to 425°F and grease a baking sheet with coconut oil or line with a Silpat or parchment paper.

⊙ Sift the flour, xanthan gum, baking powder, salt, stevia, oregano, arrowroot and tapioca starch together into the work bowl of a standing mixer.

⊙ With the mixer running on low speed, pour the cold water into the bowl slowly. Add the egg replacer/water mixture, and mix well on medium speed.

⊙ Wet hands with water, form the dough into a ball and place on the center of the greased baking sheet. Wet hands are an absolute must to prevent sticking! Wet your hands well again and, pushing down firmly on the dough, press out a 10-inch round pizza shape, working from the center out.

⊙ Bake for 9 minutes. Reduce heat to 350°, top with desired toppings (see Gluten-Free All-Veggie Pizza on page 247), and bake for another 30–35 minutes (depending on your oven), or until the edges are crispy and the bread is well done.

⊙ Be very careful moving the pizza onto a cutting board. It will be somewhat fragile, so be sure to wedge a spatula underneath it to separate it completely from the baking sheet. Use two large, flat spatulas to move the bread onto the cutting board.

ROSEMARY CAULIFLOWER "MASHED POTATOES" (COOKED VERSION)

YIELD: ABOUT 2–3 CUPS,
OR MORE DEPENDING ON CAULIFLOWER SIZE

INGREDIENTS

1 medium head cauliflower, broken into florets, stem and leaves removed

1 small clove garlic, minced

½ cup almond or coconut milk

1 Tbs. olive oil

Freshly ground black pepper, to taste

High-quality sea salt, to taste

1 tsp. dried or 1 Tbs. finely chopped rosemary

This cauliflower-based version is the same texture to enjoy as mashed potatoes, but sans the butter, whole milk and table salt that make mashed potatoes a beauty-busting food. I give it to my clients when they need that comforting texture. Try it for yourself or for a mashed potato–loving dear one.

DIRECTIONS:

⊙ Bring water to a boil and steam cauliflower in a steamer for about 6–7 minutes, until it softens.

⊙ Put the cauliflower florets in a food processor with the blade in place. Add the garlic, almond milk, olive oil, black pepper, sea salt and rosemary. Pulse long enough to achieve the desired consistency (depending on whether you are a chunky or smooth mashed potato person). Adjust seasonings to taste.

ROSEMARY CAULIFLOWER "MASHED POTATOES" (RAW VERSION)

YIELD: ABOUT 2–3 CUPS,
OR MORE DEPENDING ON CAULIFLOWER SIZE

This raw version has its advantages—namely, of course, you are consuming the raw cauliflower in all its enzyme-rich glory. However, this version is firmer and not as creamy as the cooked version. I personally love and enjoy both versions.

DIRECTIONS:

◉ Put the cauliflower in a food processor with the blade in place and chop into small pieces.

◉ Add the rest of the ingredients and process until you have the consistency you want. Adjust seasonings to taste, and serve at room temperature.

INGREDIENTS

1 medium head cauliflower, broken into florets, stem and leaves removed

1¾ cups raw pine nuts

1 very small garlic clove, minced

2 Tbs. nutritional yeast

High-quality sea salt, to taste

Freshly ground black pepper, to taste

1 tsp. dried or 1 Tbs. fresh rosemary

ITALIAN EGGPLANT CAPONATA

YIELD: ABOUT 5 CUPS

I love stocking this in my fridge. It makes great leftover snacks, and since it's all veggies you can scoop out a bit at a time to eat with gluten-free crackers or toasted millet bread. It's also an awesome accompaniment to a green salad, or as a side dish at dinner.

DIRECTIONS:

⊙ Using a steamer basket placed over boiling water, steam the eggplant, covered, for 15 minutes.

⊙ Meanwhile, heat ¼ cup of the vegetable broth in a large saucepan over medium heat and cook the onion until it is translucent. Add the celery and eggplant, and cook for another minute or two.

⊙ Add the tomatoes, capers, basil, raw apple cider vinegar and lemon juice and stir to combine.

⊙ Add the remaining cup of vegetable broth, bring to a boil, and then reduce the heat and simmer, uncovered, for about 30 minutes, until the mixture reduces down and the flavor is concentrated.

⊙ Add the stevia, sea salt and black pepper, and adjust seasonings, to taste.

⊙ Remove from heat and serve.

INGREDIENTS

6 cups peeled and diced eggplant, about 1 medium eggplant

¼ cup + 1 cup low-sodium vegetable broth

1 cup finely chopped white onion

1½ cups chopped celery, about 2 celery stalks

4 cups diced tomatoes

¼ cup drained capers

¼ cup chopped fresh basil

¼ cup raw apple cider vinegar

1 Tbs. fresh lemon juice

½ tsp. powdered stevia or about 10–12 drops liquid stevia

High-quality sea salt, to taste

Freshly ground black pepper, to taste

SIMPLE SPICED QUINOA

YIELD: ABOUT 3 CUPS

I suggest preparing a batch of this quinoa and keeping it stocked in your fridge. It will last for up to a week. You can easily double or triple the recipe.

When you're in a bind, tired or maybe just a little lazy and you would rather veg out than cook (nothing wrong with that sometimes!), you can heat this up (or not—I often eat it cold) and throw it on any kind of salad for a super-quick meal. Having items like this on hand means you can avoid resorting to processed frozen meals or takeout.

NOTE: Experiment with your favorite spices in this recipe.

INGREDIENTS

2 cups filtered water

1 cup quinoa, soaked overnight and rinsed well

1½ tsp. cumin

¼ tsp. coriander

1 Tbs. low-sodium tamari

3 Tbs. low-sodium vegetable broth

DIRECTIONS:

◉ Bring water to a boil, add quinoa and reduce heat to low. Cover and cook for about 12–15 minutes, or until quinoa is soft and fluffy. Stir in the rest of the ingredients with a fork. Adjust seasonings to taste.

HEALTHY FRENCH ONION SOUP

YIELD: 2–4 SERVINGS

INGREDIENTS

2 Tbs. + 4 cups low-sodium vegetable broth, divided

2 medium yellow onions, thinly sliced

1 garlic clove, minced

1 Tbs. raw apple cider vinegar

¼ tsp. dried thyme

High-quality sea salt, to taste

Freshly ground black pepper, to taste

2 Tbs. arrowroot starch

2–4 slices gluten-free bread, toasted with a little bit of coconut oil spread on top (optional)

Non-dairy cheese (optional)

Traditional French onion soup, which contains beef stock, white bread and cheese, demonstrates just how incredibly unhealthy soup can be. No worries, though—this vegan version has a thick, hearty base and a delicious onion flavor, which is perfect for onion soup cravings. As an option, add gluten-free bread, or you can choose to leave it out. If you are transitioning off cheese, an option is to top the bread with a non-dairy, non-soy cheese.

NOTE: The long, slow caramelizing of the onions is a crucial step that brings out the sweetness of the onions.

DIRECTIONS:

⊙ In a large soup pot, heat 2 Tbs. of vegetable broth. Gently caramelize the onions over medium heat for about 30 minutes. Do not let the temperature get too high or the onions will burn. Add the garlic, and sauté for a minute.

⊙ Add 4 cups of vegetable broth, quickly bring to a boil over high heat, and then reduce to a simmer. Add the raw apple cider vinegar, thyme, sea salt and black pepper. Continue simmering for about 40 minutes. Spoon about a cup of the broth into a bowl, and whisk in the arrowroot starch until all lumps disappear. Add the mixture to the main soup pot. Simmer for another 5 minutes. Adjust seasonings to taste.

⊙ Ladle soup into 3 or 4 ovenproof bowls and serve.

⊙ **Optional**: Preheat the oven to 400°F. Toast some gluten-free bread with a little bit of coconut oil and/or the non-dairy cheese on top, for about 5 minutes or so or until the cheese starts to melt. Remove from oven and push the bread down into each bowl of soup. Place the bowls on a baking sheet in the hot oven for another 5 minutes. Serve immediately.

ASPARAGUS AND LEEK SOUP

YIELD: ABOUT 7 CUPS

This soup is popular with my clients, who love that it has such a creamy, thick consistency without the use of any cream or milk at all. This soup is a lifesaver in the middle of the day or afternoon, as it is filling, comforting, 100 percent veggie, and totally beautifying.

DIRECTIONS:

⊙ Heat 1 Tbs. vegetable broth in a large cooking pot over medium heat, and sauté the garlic, onions and leeks. Add the celery and the asparagus, and cook for about 3–4 minutes, stirring constantly.

⊙ Add the rest of the vegetable broth and bring to a boil, then immediately reduce heat, partially cover and allow to simmer for about 25–30 minutes. Stir occasionally.

⊙ Let the soup cool, transfer to a blender and blend in batches until it's the desired smoothness. I like to leave a slightly chunky texture.

⊙ Add the soup back to the pot, and bring to a simmer. Adjust seasonings to taste.

⊙ Spoon into bowls, garnish with fresh parsley and serve.

INGREDIENTS

1 Tbs. + 3½ cups low-sodium vegetable broth, divided

3 small or 2 medium garlic cloves, minced

1½ cups chopped yellow onions

3 cups chopped leeks, both white and green parts

1 cup chopped celery

1 bunch asparagus, trimmed of tough ends and cut into 1-inch pieces

High-quality sea salt, to taste

Freshly ground black pepper, to taste

Chopped fresh parsley, as a garnish

VEGETARIAN TOM KAH THAI COCONUT SOUP

YIELD: 3–4 SERVINGS

INGREDIENTS

1¾ cups coconut milk

3 cups low-sodium vegetable broth

3 Tbs. green curry paste

2 Tbs. tamari

1 cup sliced Baby Bella mushrooms

3 cups broccoli florets

¾ cup chopped green onion

1 tsp. powdered stevia or about 15–20 drops liquid stevia

3 Tbs. fresh lime juice

1 Tbs. lime zest

Fresh whole cilantro sprigs, as a garnish

I took some Thai cooking classes while I was traveling in Thailand. It was a great experience, although my teacher, Sont, thought I was very strange indeed because I didn't want to use one little bit of animal or seafood products in my dishes, including dried shrimp, fish sauce and others that he kept telling me were "needed for taste." He did solemnly shake his head at me on more than one occasion during the classes.

Despite Sont's condolences about my shunning some of his favorite ingredients, I created this delicious, vegan version of Thai coconut soup that contains many Beauty Foods. While this and other traditional Thai dishes typically call for lemongrass, galanga root and Thai basil, I omitted them so that all the ingredients would be familiar for you and easy to find. The ethnic sections of most supermarkets now carry green curry paste. Red chili paste typically contains shrimp and fish sauce, so we leave it out. By adding the lime last, you preserve its vitamins and prevent the soup from turning sour, which is something Sont taught me that I did listen to!

DIRECTIONS:

⊙ Heat the coconut milk and vegetable broth in a large pot, along with the green curry paste and tamari. Bring to a boil, then quickly reduce heat to a simmer. Add the mushrooms, broccoli and green onion, and cook gently for 2–3 minutes, or until they are just slightly cooked, but retain most of their crispness.

⊙ Remove the pot from the heat and stir in the rest of the ingredients except the cilantro.

⊙ Ladle the soup into bowls, and top each with a generous portion of cilantro.

KALE, CARROT, PINTO BEAN AND QUINOA STEW

YIELD: 3–4 SERVINGS

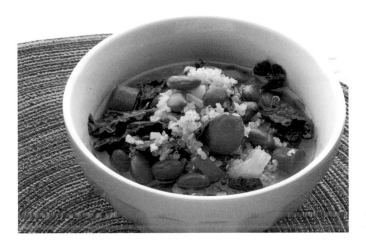

I absolutely love stews. Especially ones that contain my favorite grains, which I think go so well with the broth and vegetables. For this one, I add the kale in at the very end, so it wilts but doesn't overcook, preserving most of its nutrients.

DIRECTIONS:

⊙ Heat 1 Tbs. vegetable broth in a large saucepan over medium-high heat. Add the onions and cook until translucent. Add the garlic and cook for another minute. Be careful not to brown or burn the onions and garlic. Next, add the carrots and herbs, and cook for about 3 more minutes.

⊙ Add the remaining vegetable broth and the quinoa. Bring to a boil, then turn down the heat to low, cover, and cook for 15 minutes, until the quinoa is cooked through.

⊙ Stir in the beans, heating for about 3–5 minutes. Lastly, add the kale and simmer for about 3 more minutes, stirring frequently until kale is wilted. Cover and simmer on low for 5 more minutes. Season to taste and serve in soup bowls.

INGREDIENTS

1 Tbs. + 7 cups low-sodium vegetable broth, divided

1 cup diced white onions

2 cloves garlic, minced

2 large carrots, peeled and cut into ½-inch chunks

1 Tbs. chopped fresh marjoram

½ Tbs. minced fresh thyme

¾ tsp. minced fresh sage

1 tsp. minced fresh rosemary

½ cup quinoa

2 cups cooked pinto beans

2 cups Lacinato kale, stems removed and leaves torn into small pieces

High-quality sea salt, to taste

Freshly ground black pepper, to taste

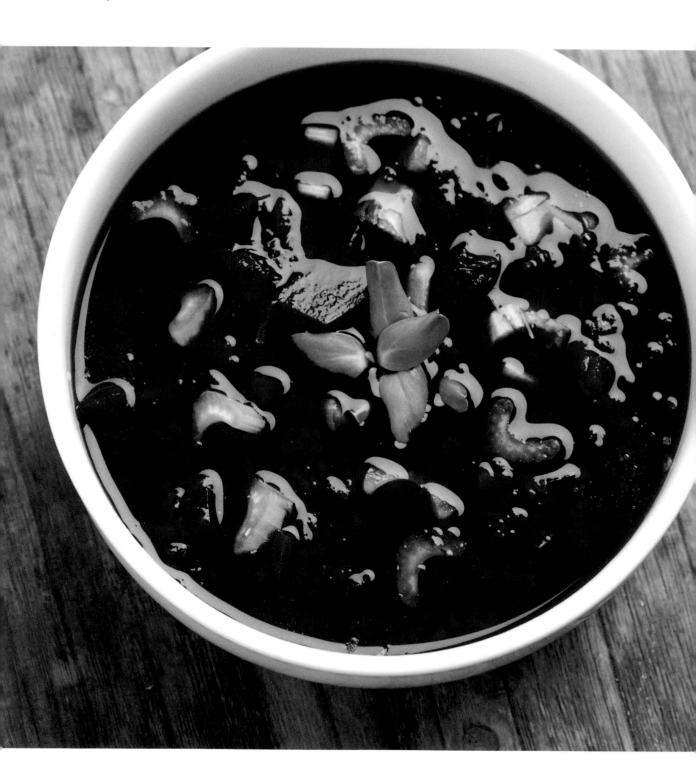

PROBIOTIC-BOOSTING POLISH BORSCHT

YIELD: 4–6 SERVINGS

I tried borscht while I was traveling through Hungary. Traditional Eastern European borscht includes kvass, which is a fermented drink made from sour black bread. Our replacement for this beneficial probiotic ingredient is a mix of two beauty foods—lemon juice and raw apple cider vinegar. Together they simulate the right sour kvass taste. Raw apple cider vinegar with the "mother," which looks like sediment and is made up of nutrients and beneficial bacteria, is fermented and extremely cleansing and nutritious (see Chapter 1), and has probiotic enhancing properties of its own.

NOTE: When peeling the beets, wear rubber gloves, an apron or something you won't mind getting stained with beet juice.

DIRECTIONS:

⊙ Heat 1 Tbs. vegetable broth in a large saucepan over low-medium heat. Add the onions and sauté until translucent. Add the garlic and sauté for a minute. Be careful not to brown or burn the onions and garlic. Then add the leeks, celery, carrots and beets. Cook for a few minutes, continuing to stir until the veggies begin to soften.

⊙ Add the remainder of the vegetable broth, bring to a boil over high heat, then reduce heat and simmer for about 25–30 minutes.

⊙ Remove the pan from the heat. Stir in the raw apple cider vinegar, lemon juice, sea salt and black pepper, and adjust seasonings.

⊙ Ladle into bowls and garnish with some freshly minced parsley. Serve immediately.

INGREDIENTS

1 Tbs. + 4 cups low-sodium vegetable broth, divided

1½ cups diced yellow onions

2 cloves garlic, minced

2 cups minced leeks

3 cups diced celery

2½ cups chopped carrots

3 cups peeled raw beets, cut into ½-inch cubes

3½ Tbs. raw apple cider vinegar

2 Tbs. fresh lemon juice

High-quality sea salt, to taste

Freshly ground black pepper, to taste

Minced parsley, to garnish

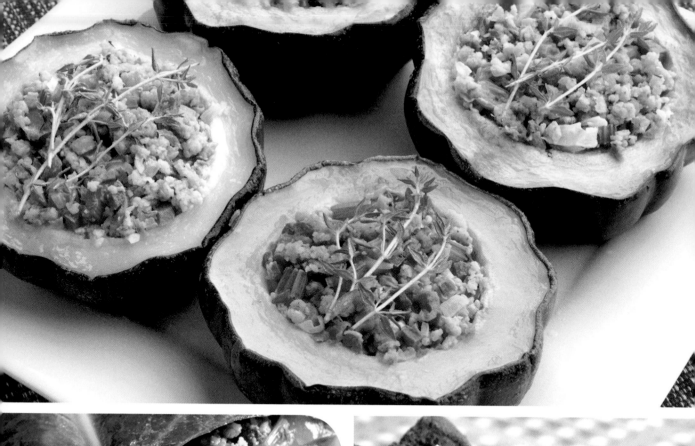

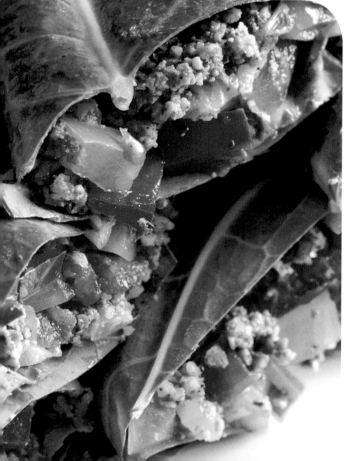

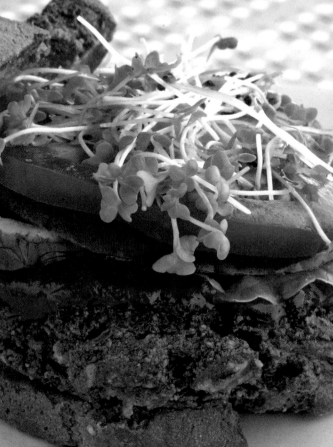

BEAUTY ENTRÉES

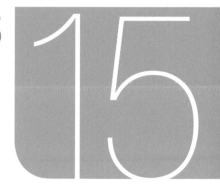

15

Note: This section includes both raw and cooked entrées. I encourage you to experiment with both types of recipes.

QUINOA, SQUASH, AVOCADO AND MICROGREEN TIMBALE STACKS

YIELD: 3 SERVINGS

INGREDIENTS

2 cups butternut squash, cubed

2 tsp. coconut oil

½ Tbs. dried rosemary, crushed

High-quality sea salt, to taste

Freshly ground black pepper, to taste

1 cup quinoa, soaked overnight and rinsed well

2 cups low-sodium vegetable broth

1½ Tbs. lime juice

2½ Tbs. minced freshly parsley

1 tsp. minced fresh basil

¼ cup finely minced purple cabbage

1 large or 2 small avocados, diced

Several handfuls of microgreens or clover sprouts, to top

Ever wonder how some dishes at a fancy restaurant come out "stacked" in a neat little tower? The secret is that the ingredients are pressed into ring molds, or ramekins, and flipped upside down on a plate for a beautiful presentation.

This dish is wonderfully balanced, because it combines the heartiness of quinoa, the raw beauty fat of avocado, the sweetness of squash and the texture of raw and nutrient-packed microgreens. The raw parsley and purple cabbage add color and a punch of extra vitamins and nutrition.

DIRECTIONS:

⊙ Preheat the oven to 375°F and grease a baking sheet with coconut oil. Toss the cubed squash with the coconut oil, rosemary and sea salt and black pepper, if desired. Bake for 20 minutes, then stir and bake for another 20 minutes.

⊙ Meanwhile, cook the quinoa in the vegetable broth for about 12 minutes, or until soft and fluffy. Add to a mixing bowl and mix in the lime juice, parsley, basil and cabbage. Season with a bit of sea salt and pepper, to your taste. Set aside.

⊙ Assemble the timbales. Take an 8-ounce ramekin, and grease lightly with coconut oil. Use one-third of the squash and pack in gently. Next add one-third of the diced avocado, and then push one-third of the quinoa mixture down into them. Press down again.

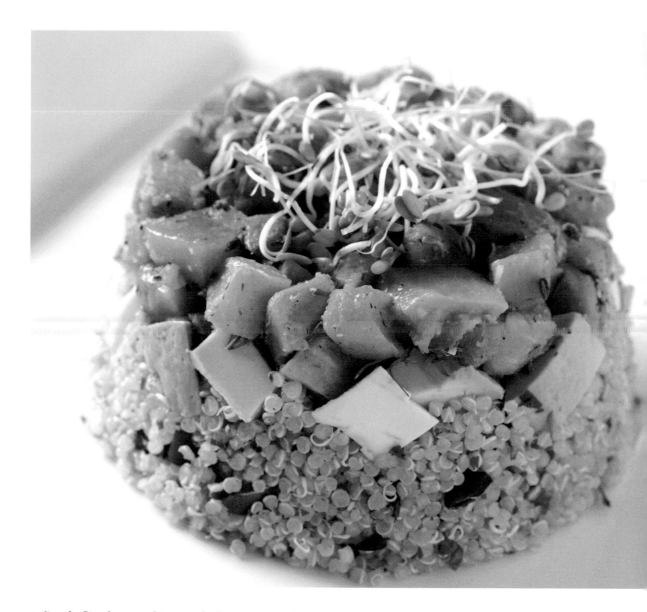

⊙ Gently flip the ramekin upside down onto a plate. Repeat
the drill three times. Top each ramekin mixture with a generous portion of microgreens or clover sprouts, arranged in a
beautiful way.

ASPARAGUS AND VEGGIE TEMPEH STIR-FRY OVER KELP NOODLES

YIELD: 4 SERVINGS

Sometimes I miss the fried noodle dishes that I once enjoyed while traveling throughout Thailand, Cambodia, Laos, Vietnam, Malaysia and the Philippines. This is a great replacement dish, and this counts as a protein dish with the tempeh. What's great is that we can still have noodles with the dish—kelp noodles—which are very low in calories (6 calories for 4 ounces) and are virtually carb-free, as they are a sea vegetable. So this is a very easily digestible dish.

NOTE: If for any reason you can't find raw kelp noodles, use rice noodles and omit the tempeh for a simpler meal with fewer food groups, and therefore easier digestion.

INGREDIENTS

8 ounces plain tempeh

1 cup + 1 Tbs. low-sodium vegetable broth, divided

¼ cup low sodium tamari

½ tsp. xanthan gum

½ tsp. powdered stevia

1 tsp. rice vinegar

1 Tbs. coconut oil

3 small garlic cloves, minced

1 cup sliced white onions

1 red or orange bell pepper, cut into 1½-inch squares

1 bunch asparagus spears (about 17–20 stalks), cut into 2-inch diagonal pieces (with tough ends discarded)

2½ cups shiitake mushrooms, sliced

24 ounces raw kelp noodles (such as Sea Tangle brand), rinsed

DIRECTIONS:

◉ Heat a pot of water to boiling, then reduce heat to low and add tempeh. Simmer for 45 minutes. Drain water, allow tempeh to cool, then cut into 1-inch chunks. Set aside.

◉ In a small bowl, whisk together 1 cup of vegetable broth, tamari, xanthan gum, stevia and rice vinegar until all lumps are worked out and set aside.

◉ Heat the coconut oil in a skillet over medium-high heat. Add tempeh, and stir-fry 4–5 minutes or until golden. The tempeh may crumble or break into smaller pieces, which is totally fine. Remove tempeh from the pan and set aside in a separate bowl.

◉ Next, heat 1 Tbs. of vegetable broth in the same pan. Add the garlic, and then the onions, and sauté for 1–2 minutes, making sure the garlic doesn't brown. Next, add the red pepper, asparagus and mushrooms to the pan, and stir-fry 4 minutes or until asparagus is crisp-tender.

◉ Add broth mixture. Bring to a boil, and gently cook for about 5 minutes, or until the sauce thickens.

◉ Add the tempeh and the raw kelp noodles, and cook for another few minutes. If you prefer a softer rather then crunchier texture in noodles, continue to cook for a few minutes longer in the sauce. Serve in individual bowls.

GLUTEN-FREE VEGAN LASAGNA SUPREME

YIELD: 8 SERVINGS

This is a hearty dish that is great after a huge salad. If you are transitioning or if you are making this for someone who usually eats heavier foods, you can certainly add some non-dairy, non-soy cheese to your lasagna. Don't forget to take your digestive enzymes before eating!

INGREDIENTS

12–14 ounces gluten-free lasagna noodles, cooked, drained and set to the side (some brown rice, gluten-free pastas don't have to be precooked)

6 cups broccoli, chopped into very small florets

5 cups chopped spinach

High-quality sea salt, to taste

Freshly ground black pepper, to taste

32 ounces Homemade Bella Marinara (see page 185)

Soy-free vegan cheese (optional)

DIRECTIONS:

⊙ Cook gluten-free lasagna noodles in a large pot of boiling water for 10 minutes, or until al dente. Drain and set aside. Omit this step for gluten-free noodles that don't need to be precooked.

⊙ Boil some water in a pot, and steam the broccoli and spinach in a steamer until the broccoli is softened and the spinach is wilted—about 4 minutes or so. Add a little sea salt and freshly ground black pepper, just to give the veggies a bit of flavor. Preheat the oven to 350°F.

⊙ In a 9 x 13 inch baking dish, apply a thin layer of marinara sauce to cover entire dish. Then layer one-third of the noodles, one-third of the marinara sauce, one-third of the broccoli and spinach, and then one-third of the vegan cheese, if you choose to use it. Repeat the layers with the remaining ingredients.

⊙ Cover in foil lined with parchment paper and bake in a pre-heated oven for about 60 minutes. (Cooking time depends on the type of gluten-free pasta you use, as well as your oven. Follow directions on the box.) Uncover and bake another 5 minutes. Let stand for 5–10 minutes before serving.

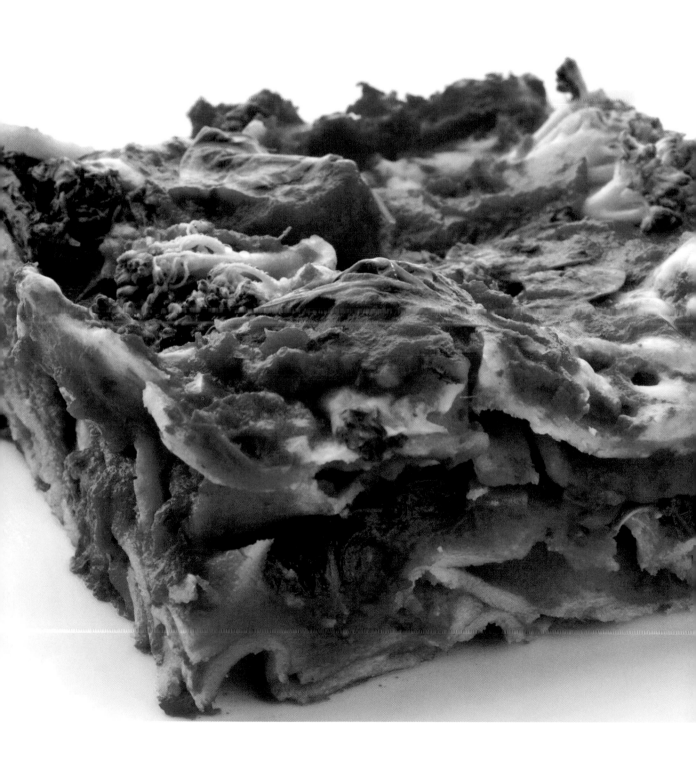

PORTOBELLO MUSHROOM BURGERS

YIELD: ABOUT 8 BURGERS

INGREDIENTS

4 portobello mushroom caps, or about 8 ounces, diced

½ cup chopped fresh parsley

1 Tbs. low-sodium vegetable broth

1 clove garlic, minced

¾ cup finely chopped white onions

½ cup finely chopped celery

2½ Tbs. organic ketchup (If you can't find organic ketchup, omit this. Do not use regular ketchup.)

½ Tbs. finely chopped fresh thyme

1 tsp. finely chopped fresh oregano

½ tsp. finely chopped fresh sage

1 Tbs. low-sodium tamari

1 tsp. high-quality sea salt

2 cups Gluten-Free Bread Crumbs (see page 216)

Romaine lettuce hearts, collard green wraps or sliced gluten-free bread, for serving

It irks me that most commercial veggie burgers contain soy, wheat or both. This version has neither. One of my clients told me this is the best veggie burger she ever had. [Blush.] I'm excited to share it with you here.

DIRECTIONS:

⊙ In a food processor with the chopping blade in place, process the mushrooms and parsley until finely minced. Scrape the mixture into a large mixing bowl.

⊙ In a skillet over low-medium heat, heat the vegetable broth and cook the garlic and onions for a few minutes until translucent. Add the celery and cook for another minute.

⊙ Add the vegetables to the mixing bowl with the mushroom-parsley mixture. Add the organic ketchup, and the herbs and seasonings. Finally, add the bread crumbs. Mix well and adjust seasoning to taste.

⊙ Refrigerate to cool for at least 45 minutes or longer, so it becomes easier to form the mixture into patties.

⊙ Preheat the oven to 350°F.

⊙ Moisten your hands with a little water, and form patties.

⊙ Line a baking sheet with parchment paper and bake the patties for 30 minutes or until they are cooked through.

⊙ Serve on romaine lettuce hearts, in collard green wraps or on gluten-free bread.

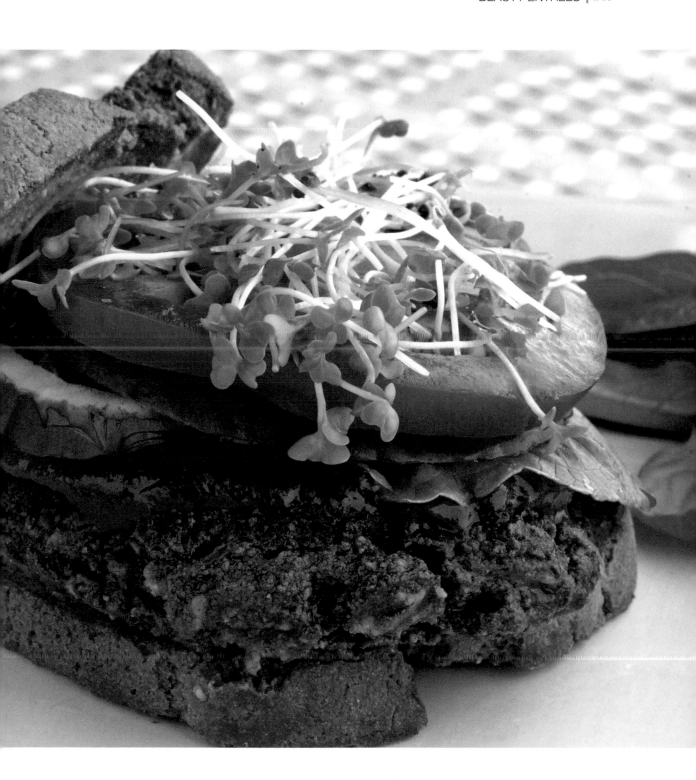

CUMIN CHILI CHICKPEA BURGERS

YIELD: 6 BURGERS

This makes for a solid, tasty burger when you're in the mood for something substantial. Also great for husbands and boyfriends! I often eat these burgers with big lettuce leaves, in collard green wraps or sliced over a salad instead of bread, as they are fairly dense.

INGREDIENTS

2 cups cooked chickpeas

1¼ cups Gluten-Free Bread Crumbs (see page 216)

1 tsp. chili powder

½ tsp. cumin

3 Tbs. low sodium tamari

2 Tbs. organic ketchup (If you can't find organic ketchup, omit this. Do not use regular ketchup.)

1 Tbs. low-sodium vegetable broth

1 clove garlic, finely minced or pressed

2 Tbs. minced shallots

1½ Tbs. finely minced parsley

DIRECTIONS:

⊙ Place the chickpeas in the food processor and process, leaving the mixture somewhat chunky. Place in a large mixing bowl.

⊙ Add the bread crumbs, chili powder, cumin, tamari and organic ketchup. Mix well and set aside.

⊙ In a large skillet, heat the vegetable broth and cook the garlic and shallots until they are translucent, about 3 minutes. Add to the mixture in the bowl. Stir in the parsley. Allow the mixture to cool in the fridge for at least half an hour. Once it has cooled, form patties in your hands.

⊙ Preheat the oven to 350°F.

⊙ Line a baking sheet with parchment paper and bake the patties for 30 minutes or until they are cooked through.

SPANISH MILLET PAELLA

YIELD: 6–8 SERVINGS

Dishes similar to paella are a traditional part of my family's heritage, and I remember as a child loving the flavor of the yellow rice or noodles and veggies, but picking around the meat and seafood. This dish has the familiar flavors I still love, and the millet is a much better beauty substitute for the yellow rice.

DIRECTIONS:

⊙ Preprep: Soak the millet the night before then rinse well before beginning the recipe.

⊙ Heat ¼ cup vegetable broth over low-medium heat in a large pot and add the saffron. When the saffron begins to brown slightly, add the onions, garlic and scallions, and sauté gently for a few moments. Next, add the carrots, pepper and millet, and cook the mixture for a few moments, stirring to distribute the ingredients evenly throughout the millet.

⊙ Add 5 cups of vegetable stock and reduce heat to medium-low. Cook the mixture for about 18 minutes, or until the millet has softened somewhat. Be sure to stir occasionally.

⊙ Stir in tomatoes and snap peas. Mix them in, and then cover the pot and cook for about 5 minutes, until the millet is al dente and the snap peas have softened a bit. The paella should retain a creamy, risotto-like texture from the vegetable broth. Add sea salt and adjust to taste, and serve hot.

INGREDIENTS

2 cups millet

¼ cup + 5 cups low-sodium vegetable broth, divided

A few saffron threads

1 cup diced yellow onion

2 cloves garlic, minced

½ cup diced scallions

2 carrots, peeled and diced

1 medium red bell pepper, diced

1 cup diced fresh tomatoes

½ pound sugar snap peas

High-quality sea salt, to taste

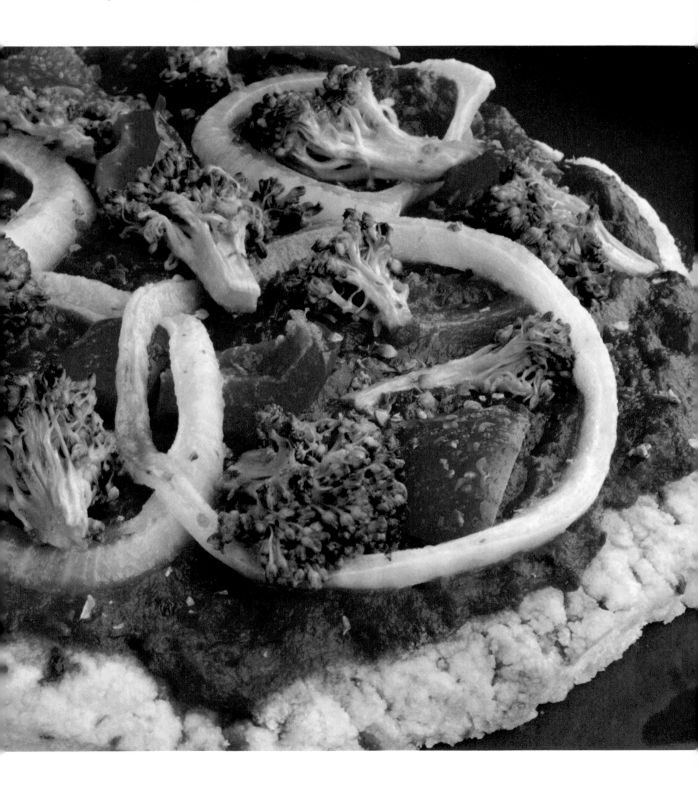

GLUTEN-FREE ALL-VEGGIE PIZZA

YIELD: TWO 10-INCH PIZZAS

Once you get the hang of the Miracle Gluten-Free Vegan Pizza Dough, you'll love this tasty pizza. It makes a fairly thick crust, so you will not need to eat as much as you do with regular pizza. If you're transitioning or making this for someone who is used to heavier food, you can include some kind of non-dairy cheese, if you like.

DIRECTIONS:

◉ Preheat the oven to 350°F. Grease a large baking sheet with some coconut oil.

◉ Heat the vegetable broth in a skillet over medium heat and add the onions. Cook the onions, stirring constantly and partly caramelizing them for about 5 minutes. Watch carefully to make sure they don't burn.

◉ Next, add the red pepper and broccoli to the skillet, and cook for only another 3 minutes and remove from the heat. Add some more vegetable broth, if needed. The red pepper and broccoli should still be crisp. Season with sea salt and black pepper to taste.

◉ Place the 2 pizza dough breads on the baking sheet, and spread the marinara sauce in an even layer over each of the breads, and then spoon the vegetable mixture evenly over the breads. Sprinkle some oregano over the top.

◉ Bake the breads for about 35 minutes, as per the partly baked Miracle Gluten-Free Vegan Pizza Dough recipe (see page 218), or if the dough you are using is already cooked, bake for 10–15 minutes, or until the edges of the bread are crisp and lightly browned. Top with oregano.

INGREDIENTS

Coconut oil, for oiling pan

2 Tbs. low-sodium vegetable broth

1 cup thinly sliced yellow onions

1 red pepper, cored, seeded and chopped into ½-inch squares

1 cup broccoli florets

High-quality sea salt, to taste

Freshly ground black pepper, to taste

2 batches Miracle Gluten-Free Vegan Pizza Dough, (see page 218) or other pizza crusts, preferably gluten-free

1½ cups Homemade Bella Marinara (see page 185)

Dried or freshly minced oregano, for topping

JENNA'S BAKED FALAFEL

YIELD: ABOUT 15 BALLS

I normally avoid falafel because it is deep-fried. When I was working as the chef and nutritionist for the lead actor on a movie set, my friend Jenna, who loves Middle Eastern food, inspired me to experiment with making her a vegan, gluten-free, baked falafel, and she loved it! This baked version will supply those falafel flavors, but without all that cooked oil.

INGREDIENTS

Coconut oil, for oiling pan and hands

2 cups cooked chickpeas

1 Tbs. vegetable broth

1 cup finely chopped onions

2 small garlic cloves, minced

3 Tbs. chopped fresh parsley

1 Tbs. chopped fresh cilantro

1 tsp. lemon juice

1 tsp. olive oil

1 tsp. coriander

1 tsp. cumin

⅛ tsp. cayenne pepper

2 Tbs. chickpea flour

1 tsp. baking powder

½ tsp. high-quality sea salt

¼ tsp. freshly ground black pepper

Oil-Free Garlic, Raw Apple Cider Vinegar, Tahini and Almond Butter Dressing (see page 186)

DIRECTIONS:

◉ Preheat the oven to 375°F. Oil a baking sheet with coconut oil or use a Silpat or parchment paper to line the sheet.

◉ Mash the chickpeas in a food processor, or place the chickpeas in a medium-sized bowl and smash with a fork. Place into a large mixing bowl.

◉ Heat the vegetable broth in a small pan and gently cook the onions for a few minutes until translucent. Add the garlic and cook for another minute. Add to the mixing bowl.

◉ Add the rest of the ingredients, except dressing, and mix well. Put a small amount of coconut oil on your hands, and form the mixture into small balls, about the size of a Ping-Pong ball. Place onto the oiled baking pan.

◉ Bake for about 22 minutes, then flip with a spatula and bake on the other side for another 22 minutes, or until the part touching the pan begins to slightly brown.

◉ Serve in preferably gluten-free or sprouted grain pita pockets or over a green salad, with Raw Chickpea-Less Hummus from *The Beauty Detox Solution* or Oil-Free Garlic, Raw Apple Cider Vinegar, Tahini and Almond Butter Dressing (page 186), along with tomatoes, lettuce and/or cucumbers.

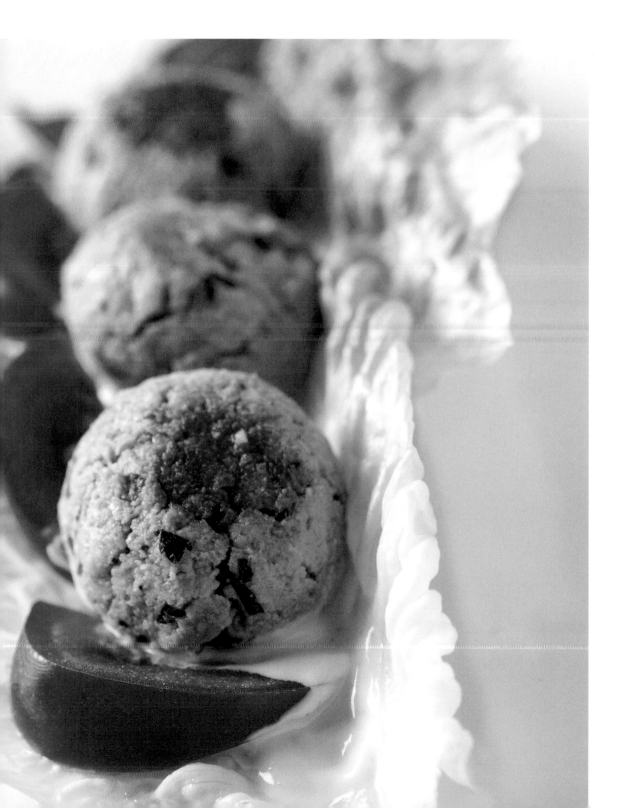

SHIVA-SHAKTI DAAL

YIELD: 4–6 SERVINGS

INGREDIENTS

1 cup dried red lentils, rinsed and picked over

1 Tbs. + 4 cups low-sodium vegetable broth, divided

2 cloves garlic, finely chopped

1 cup finely chopped white onions

1 Tsp. finely chopped fresh ginger

1 tsp. cumin

1 tsp. coriander

¾ tsp. turmeric

¼ tsp. powdered cardamom

¼ tsp. cinnamon

Cooked quinoa, for serving

Whenever I eat daal, which is an Indian lentil stew, I think of Kashmir, in northern India. When I was traveling in that part of the world, I arrived very late one evening at a guesthouse. The caretaker insisted on making me daal and basmati rice, which we ate together sitting on little rugs on the floor and with no utensils. In my famished state, it tasted about as good as anything I had ever eaten. After that, I ate daal and rice in many different variations across different regions I journeyed to for the three months I was in India. It still occupies a special place in my heart. I like to eat the daal plain or over quinoa. Be sure to eat a green salad first.

DIRECTIONS:

⊙ Preprep: Rinse the lentils well, picking out any black or discolored pieces. Soak lentils in spring or filtered water overnight.

⊙ Heat 1 Tbs. of vegetable broth in a large saucepan over medium-high heat. Add the garlic, white onions and ginger, and sauté for a few minutes, until the onions become translucent. Be careful not to burn or brown them.

⊙ Add the rest of the vegetable broth, and bring to a boil. Reduce heat to low, and add the lentils.

⊙ Stir in the spices, and cook until the lentils are tender, stirring occasionally, for about 20 minutes. Serve over quinoa, or eat on its own.

SESAME SEED–TEMPEH GORILLA WRAPS

YIELD: 4–6 FULL WRAPS OR 8–12 HALVES,
DEPENDING ON HOW BIG THE COLLARD LEAVES ARE

I coined the term *gorilla wraps,* because whole collard greens look sturdy enough to be growing in the jungle, and remind me of something a gorilla could feast on. I make variations of Gorilla Wraps for my clients often. They are a great way to get greens in besides a salad, and feel like you're eating a fun type of sandwich, since you can pick it up. This version, which contains tempeh, is a nice, hearty variety—one I like to work into the rotation occasionally.

DIRECTIONS:

⊙ Bring a large pot of water to the boil. Add tempeh, lower the heat and simmer for about 45 minutes. Remove and drain in a colander. Once cooled, cut into half-inch squares.

⊙ Heat coconut oil over medium-high heat in a large skillet, add the garlic and scallion, and sauté for a minute. Add the grated ginger, reduce the heat and cook for another 2 minutes.

⊙ Add the tempeh, and stir to mix. Pour the tamari and raw apple cider vinegar over the tempeh as you continue to stir. The tempeh will start to brown. Add the red pepper flakes and the basil and cook for another minute. Turn off the heat and toss in the sesame oil and sesame seeds. Stir to mix. They shouldn't be cooked.

⊙ Spoon a small mixture down the middle of each collard green and wrap, burrito-style, folding the ends in. Slice diagonally halfway through and serve.

INGREDIENTS

8 ounces tempeh, cubed into ½-inch pieces

1½ Tbs. coconut oil

1 garlic clove, minced

1 cup chopped scallion, white and green parts

¾ Tbs. grated ginger

1 Tbs. low-sodium tamari

1 tsp. raw apple cider vinegar

½ tsp. red pepper flakes

½ cup fresh basil

2 tsp. sesame oil

1½ Tbs. sesame seeds

1 bunch collard greens, washed, dried and with thick stem cut off, about 2 inches from the edge of the leaf (Try to find collards that are free of holes, to prevent the mixture from falling through.)

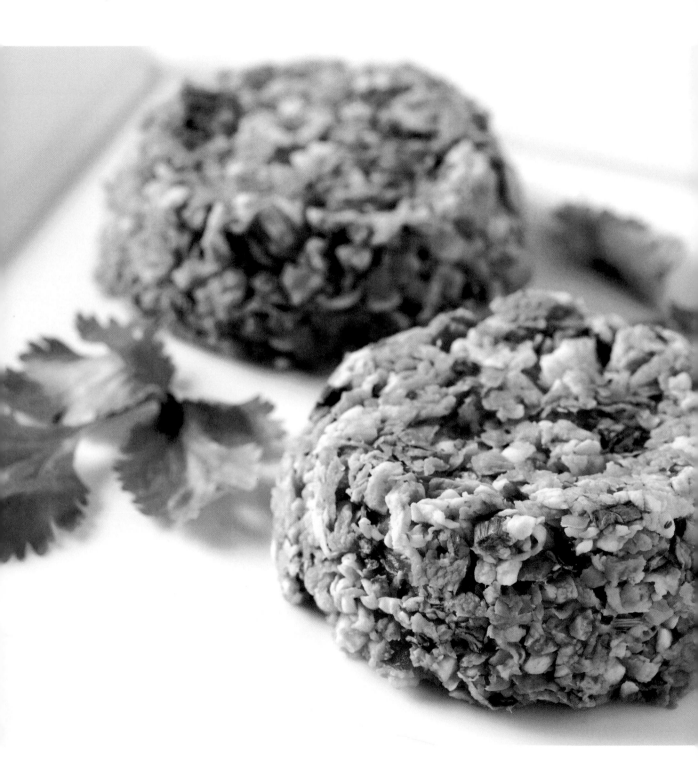

SOUTHWESTERN SAVORY ROOT VEGETABLE LATKES

YIELD: 6 LATKES

Latkes are potato pancakes that are usually made with potatoes and wheat flour and then deep-fried. This gluten-free, vegan version has a base of beautifying sweet potatoes and yams, and are packed with vegetables. Much healthier than the original! I like to serve them topped with salsa, alongside a salad, for a satisfying lunch or dinner.

DIRECTIONS:

⊙ Preheat the oven to 350°F and grease a baking sheet with some coconut oil, or lay some parchment paper down on a baking sheet.

⊙ In a large bowl, mix together the grated sweet potato, grated yam, cayenne pepper, chili powder, cumin and sea salt.

⊙ Next, add the scallions, spinach and tomatoes, and mix well. Moisten hands with a little coconut oil and form pancake patties, about 4 inches in diameter. Place them on the baking sheet. Bake for 40 minutes, or until the latkes become firm and cook through. Top with salsa.

INGREDIENTS

Coconut oil, for oiling pan and moistening hands

2½ cups grated sweet potato

2½ cups grated yam

¼ tsp. cayenne pepper

½ tsp. chili powder

½ tsp. cumin

1 tsp. high quality sea salt

½ cup chopped scallions

1 cup chopped spinach

¾ cup diced tomatoes

Salsa, for topping

GREEN SPRING VEGETABLE RISOTTO

YIELD: 5–6 SERVINGS

This is a vegan, butterless and Parmesan cheese-less version of risotto with a wonderful creamy texture. Because of the consistency of brown rice, it requires more vegetable broth and cooking time than risotto, which uses other rice varieties, such as Arborio. It's key to eat a large green salad before this dish, to help control portion size.

INGREDIENTS

1 pound asparagus, woody ends trimmed off about 2 inches from bottom, and cut into 1-inch pieces

1 Tbs. + 8 cups low-sodium vegetable broth, divided

1 bunch scallions, chopped

2 cups short-grain brown rice

1 Tbs. fresh lemon juice

3 Tbs. nutritional yeast

High-quality sea salt, to taste

Freshly ground black pepper, to taste

DIRECTIONS:

⊙ Cook the asparagus in a steamer until softened, about 6–7 minutes.

⊙ In a separate saucepan, bring the 8 cups of vegetable broth to a boil, then reduce immediately to a simmer.

⊙ Meanwhile, heat 1 Tbs. vegetable broth in a large saucepan, and begin to cook the scallions. Add the brown rice, and cook over medium heat for 2 minutes, stirring constantly.

⊙ Add the lemon juice to the rice, and stir until it is absorbed.

⊙ Add 2 cups of the broth mixture to the rice and green onion mixture, stirring constantly until the liquid is absorbed. Continue adding the broth, one ladle at a time, to the mixture, and keep stirring.

⊙ When the liquid is mostly absorbed and the rice is tender but still firm, remove from heat. This takes about 40–45 minutes or longer, depending on the exact variety of brown rice you are using.

⊙ Stir in the steamed asparagus. Add the nutritional yeast, sea salt and black pepper to suit your taste and serve immediately.

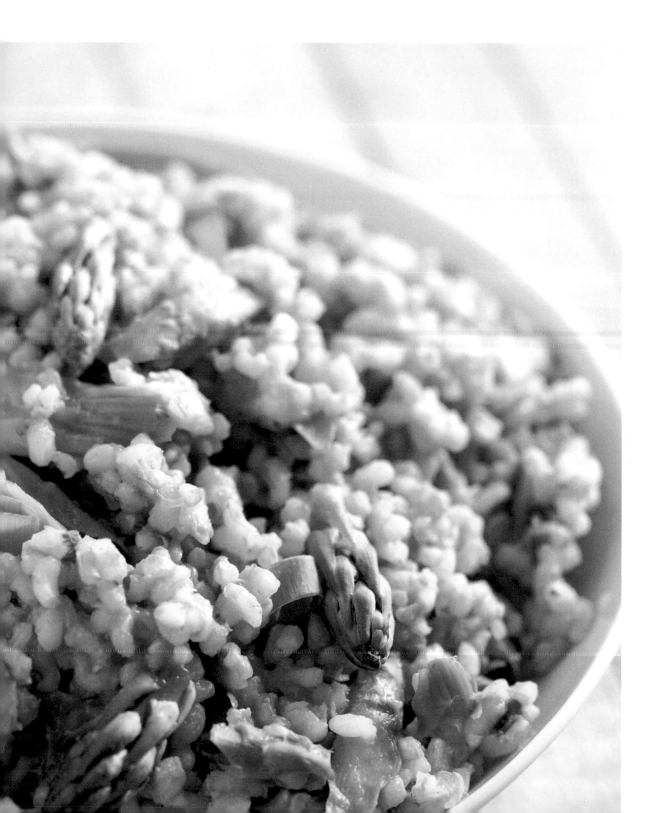

BAKED STUFFED VEGGIE EGGPLANT

YIELD: 4 SERVINGS

When you use larger eggplants, this makes a great entrée for a lighter dinner. You can also serve it with a vegetable or two on the side. If you use smaller eggplants, it makes a beautiful appetizer for a dinner party, served, of course, after a raw green salad.

INGREDIENTS

2 medium eggplants
(6–7 inches long each)

Coconut oil, for coating pan

1 Tbs. low-sodium vegetable broth

2 cloves garlic, minced

1 cup diced white onions

2 cups diced tomatoes

High-quality sea salt,
to taste

Freshly ground black pepper,
to taste

¼ tsp. dried oregano

2½ cups Gluten-Free Bread Crumbs
(see page 216)

1 tsp. olive oil

4 thin tomato slices, reserved

Fresh parsley, for garnish

DIRECTIONS:

⊙ Cut each eggplant in half. Scoop out the seeds from the center and discard. Then, with a paring knife, cut in toward the middle and carefully pull out the eggplant pulp, leaving about half an inch on the sides of the eggplant. Cut the pulp up into small half-inch or smaller pieces, and place in a bowl. Set aside.

⊙ Preheat the oven to 350°F.

⊙ Heat a large saucepan with enough coconut oil to lightly coat the bottom. Cook the eggplant shells for about 3 minutes, cut side down, to soften, and then flip them over to cook for another 3 minutes. Place in a baking pan, just big enough to hold them, with the open side face up.

⊙ Meanwhile, heat the vegetable broth over medium heat, and cook the garlic and white onions for a minute. Add the diced tomatoes and chopped pieces of eggplant, as well as the sea salt, black pepper and oregano. Lower the heat and cook for a few more moments to bring out the flavors. The liquid from the tomato and eggplant will start to come out, creating additional moistness to the mixture.

⊙ Turn off the heat and stir in the bread crumbs. Adjust seasonings, to taste. Add a tiny amount of olive oil, to help moisten the mixture. Spoon into the eggplant shells, packing it in well. Cover each eggplant half with the thinly sliced tomatoes.

⊙ Line some foil with parchment paper and tuck the ends in so that no foil can touch your eggplants. Cover the eggplants with the parchment paper foil covering and bake the stuffed eggplants for 45 minutes. Remove from the oven and garnish with some fresh parsley.

STUFFED ACORN SQUASH

YIELD: 4 SERVINGS

INGREDIENTS

2 acorn squash

Coconut oil, for rubbing on squash

2 cloves garlic, minced

½ tsp. high-quality sea salt

½ Tbs. vegetable broth

1 cup chopped onions

2 cloves garlic

2 celery stalks, diced

2 medium carrots, diced

1 tsp. fresh thyme leaves

1 tsp. minced fresh sage

1 tsp. minced fresh oregano

1½ tsp. raw apple cider vinegar

1 cup Gluten-Free Bread Crumbs (see page 216)

Freshly ground black pepper, to taste

Fresh sprigs of thyme, for garnish

This is a favorite recipe of Drew, a dear friend and client, whom I love very much. I hope you like it, too.

DIRECTIONS:

⊙ Line a baking pan with parchment paper.

⊙ Cut squash in half and remove seeds. Rub a little coconut oil over all the orange squash skin, as well as the minced garlic and a bit of sea salt. Bake, cut side up on the baking pan, at 350°F for 30 minutes. If the squash halves are wobbly on the baking pan, shave a bit from the bottom of each squash half, so each half can lay flat.

⊙ Meanwhile, heat the vegetable broth in a sauté pan. Add the onions and cook for a few minutes until they become translucent, then add the garlic, and cook for another minute. Next, add the celery and carrots. Sauté until they are soft. Add the herbs, and then the raw apple cider vinegar.

⊙ Add the bread crumbs, and stir for 2 minutes. Stir in sea salt and black pepper, and adjust seasonings to taste. Remove mixture from the heat.

⊙ Add the stuffing to cavities of the squash, mounding as needed, and bake, covered with parchment paper tucked into aluminum foil, for another 20 minutes. To create a crunchy top, remove the foil and bake for an additional 15 minutes. Lay a few sprigs of fresh thyme across each squash, to garnish, and serve.

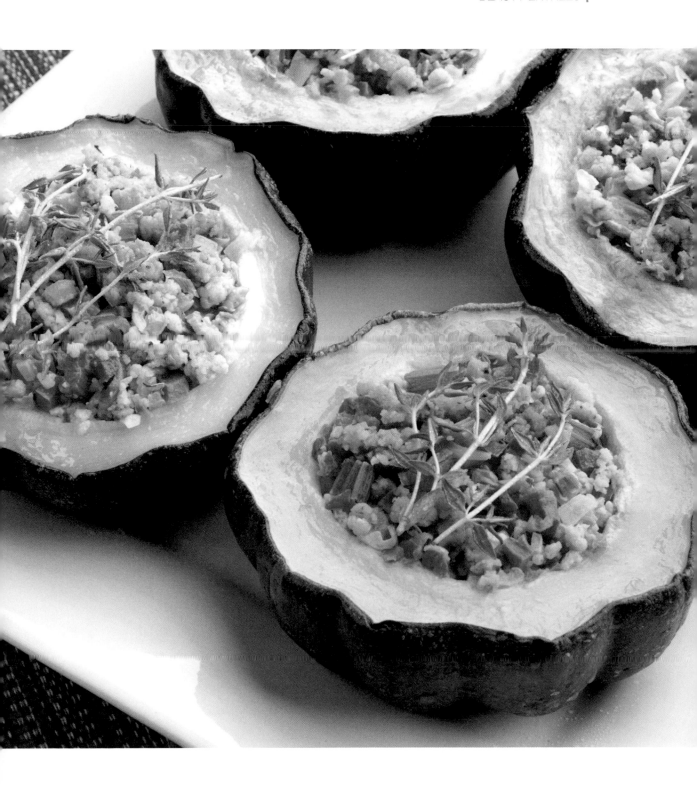

SWEET POTATO SHEPHERD'S PIE

YIELD: 11–12 SERVINGS

INGREDIENTS

Coconut oil, for greasing pan

3 large sweet potatoes, chopped into thirds (peel the sweet potatoes, if you like)

½ cup almond milk

High-quality sea salt, to taste

Freshly ground black pepper, to taste

2 Tbs. + ½ cup low-sodium vegetable broth, divided

1 cup chopped onions

1 clove garlic, minced

1 cup chopped celery

1¼ cups peeled and diced carrots

1 cup fresh (preferably) or frozen peas

Kernels from 2 ears of fresh organic corn

1¼ tsp. fresh thyme leaves

2 tsp. finely minced fresh rosemary

1 Tbs. arrowroot starch

¼ cup Ener-G egg replacer, mixed with ¾ cup very hot water

Nutmeg (optional)

This is a hearty dish that my client Channing loves. Ladies, this may be a good one for your husbands, boyfriends or brothers to show them that eating a meatless dish can, in fact, fill you up. I like to keep the skin on the sweet potatoes for maximum nutrition.

DIRECTIONS:

⊙ Lightly grease a 2-quart glass casserole dish with coconut oil.

⊙ In a large saucepan, bring enough water to a boil to cover sweet potatoes completely, and add the sweet potatoes. Reduce the heat, and simmer for about 30 minutes, or until softened.

⊙ Drain sweet potatoes and place in a large mixing bowl; mash lightly. Add the almond milk. Blend the potato mixture with an electric hand mixer set to medium until smooth and fluffy, about 2 minutes. Season with sea salt and black pepper. Set aside.

⊙ Heat 2 Tbs. of vegetable broth in a large skillet over medium heat. Cook the onions over medium-low heat until translucent, then add the garlic and cook for another minute. Add the celery, carrots, peas, corn, thyme and rosemary. Increase the heat to medium-high. In a small bowl, whisk together the rest of the vegetable broth and arrowroot until smooth, and add to the skillet. When the mixture gets close to boiling, immediately reduce heat. Add sea salt and black pepper, and season to taste. Remove from heat. Stir in the egg replacer/water combination.

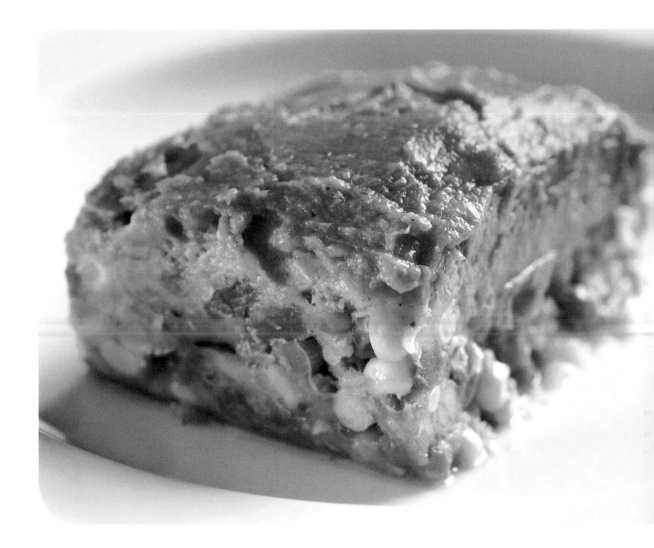

◉ Pour the veggie mixture into the bottom of the prepared casserole dish, spreading it evenly across the bottom. Spoon the sweet potato mixture over the vegetables, spreading to cover all the way to the edges of the dish. Sprinkle the top with nutmeg, if desired.

◉ Bake in a preheated 375°F oven until the top is slightly browned, about 40 minutes. Allow to rest 20 minutes or more before serving.

YIN-YANG MEAL: BAKED SQUASH, STEAMED KALE AND QUINOA PILAF

YIELD: 3–4 SERVINGS

INGREDIENTS

Coconut oil, for greasing pan

1 large butternut squash, or 2 smaller ones

Low-sodium tarami

1 large bunch Lacinato kale, or 2 smaller bunches, chopped or torn; stems optional

Whole dulse leaves or flakes (optional)

High-quality sea salt (optional), to taste

1 tsp. freshly squeezed lime juice

2 Tbs. low-sodium vegetable broth

½ cup scallions, diced

1 garlic clove, minced

1½ cups cooked quinoa

This balanced dish is one of my favorite kinds of meals: the pairing of cooked green veggies and a Beauty Detox starch, or in this case two, which can be digested well together. This dish is reminiscent of a plate I would order in a macrobiotic restaurant, except I swapped the classic macrobiotic staple of brown rice for quinoa. I love to serve this dish beautifully presented in separate mounds, then eat a bite with some of all three components together in a perfect balance. I love when foods—and life—are balanced, don't you?

DIRECTIONS:

⊙ Preprep: Soak quinoa overnight in water and rinse well before cooking.

BAKED SQUASH

⊙ Preheat the oven to 375°F and grease a baking sheet with coconut oil, or use a Silpat or parchment paper to line the sheet.

⊙ Slice the butternut squash in half and scoop out the seeds and inner stringy part. Place sliced side down on the baking sheet and bake for 45 minutes or until cooked through.

⊙ Cut each squash into quarters, and mound on one-third of each plate. Serve plain, or rub a little bit of tamari, as desired, into the squash.

STEAMED KALE

◉ Place kale in a pot with a steamer and add an inch of water to the pot. Cover the pot with a lid and steam for a few minutes. Toss with whole dulse leaves or flakes for added flavor or add a little bit of high-quality sea salt, if desired. Add in the lime juice and toss through. Arrange the kale over one-third of the plate.

QUINOA PILAF

◉ Heat the vegetable broth in a saucepan. Add the scallions and cook over medium heat until translucent. Add the garlic, and cook for another minute.

◉ Add the cooked quinoa, and stir everything together in the pan. Add a tablespoon or so of tamari as desired, for flavor.

◉ Pack into a small bowl or ramekin greased with a little coconut oil and push down firmly to make a solid mass. Invert the bowl over the remaining third of the plate, tapping on the bowl until it releases its contents.

BLACK BEAN BURRITOS WITH SPICY RED SAUCE

YIELD: 4 BURRITOS

This is especially great plane food or whenever you're in the mood for some Mexican flavors. You can adjust the spice levels to be more mild, so it can be a great dish to serve to your kids as well. Ideally, serve these after or alongside a large chopped romaine salad.

DIRECTIONS:

⊙ Grease an 8 x 8 inch baking pan with some coconut oil.

⊙ In a medium cooking pot, bring 2 cups vegetable broth to a boil, then reduce heat to a simmer. Add the brown rice, and cook for about 45 minutes, or until the rice is cooked al dente. Add the beans and seasonings into the pot, and adjust to taste. Set aside.

⊙ Heat the remaining 1 Tbs. vegetable broth in a large saucepan. Sauté the onion until it becomes translucent, then add the garlic. Cook for 1 more minute. Add the spinach and stir until it wilts. Add the red peppers, and cook for another 2 minutes. Season the veggies with a little sea salt and black pepper.

⊙ Place a quarter of the rice and bean mixture and a quarter of the veggies in the middle of one of the tortillas and fold in toward the middle, tucking the edges in at the same time. Place in the baking pan, with the folded edge facing down. Repeat until the mixture has been spread across all four burritos.

BASE INGREDIENTS

Coconut oil, for greasing pan

2 cups + 1 Tbs. low-sodium vegetable broth, divided

1 cup dry brown rice, soaked overnight and rinsed thoroughly

2 cups cooked black beans

½ tsp. chili powder

⅛ tsp. coriander

½ tsp. cumin

Pinch of cayenne pepper (or more, if you are a spicy person!)

High-quality sea salt, to taste

Freshly ground black pepper, to taste

1 small onion, sliced

1 clove garlic, minced

4 cups coarsely chopped spinach, stems removed, or baby spinach leaves

2 small red peppers, cored, seeded and sliced

4 brown rice or organic corn tortillas (spelt tortillas are an option, too, but note that spelt does contain gluten)

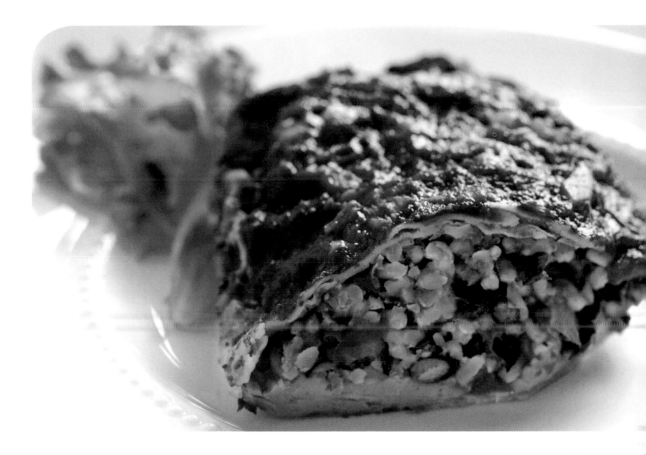

To make the spicy red sauce: Using the same saucepan, heat 1 Tbs. vegetable broth over medium heat, and then cook the onion and garlic until translucent. Add the rest of the vegetable broth, tomato paste, chili powder, cumin, coriander and cayenne pepper. Bring to a boil, then quickly reduce heat and simmer for about 5 minutes. Pour about $\frac{1}{4}$ of the sauce over each burrito.

Cover the baking pan in foil lined with parchment paper and bake in a preheated 350°F oven for about 30 minutes.

RED SAUCE INGREDIENTS

1 Tbs. + 1 cup low-sodium vegetable broth

¼ cup chopped onion

1 clove garlic, minced

¼ cup tomato paste from a glass container

1 tsp. chili powder

½ tsp. cumin

¼ tsp. ground coriander

Pinch cayenne pepper

SMOKY TEMPEH OVER SAUTÉED BROCCOLI RABE

YIELD: 4 SERVINGS

INGREDIENTS

1 large bay leaf

¼ cup + ⅓ cup low-sodium tamari, divided

16 ounces tempeh (2 standard packages)

3 Tbs. raw coconut nectar (or maple syrup)

1 Tbs. raw apple cider vinegar

1 Tbs. fresh lemon juice, plus extra to squeeze over broccoli rabe

1½–2 pounds broccoli rabe, with the last few inches of tough ends trimmed off

1 Tbs. coconut oil

2 Tbs. low-sodium vegetable broth

2 garlic cloves, minced finely

High-quality sea salt, to taste

Freshly ground black pepper, to taste

When I eat tempeh, I always eat a large green salad first, then pair it with lots of greens, like the delicious broccoli rabe in this dish. This helps control portions and improves the digestion of the tempeh, which is a pretty dense, concentrated food.

DIRECTIONS:

⊙ Bring 6 cups of water, the bay leaf, and ¼ cup tamari to a boil in a large pot. Reduce the heat, add the tempeh, and simmer for 45 minutes.

⊙ Meanwhile, in a large mixing bowl, mix together the remaining ⅓ cup tamari, coconut nectar or maple syrup, raw apple cider vinegar and lemon juice.

⊙ Cut the tempeh into four equal-sized pieces, and place in the mixing bowl to marinade in the liquid for at least 45 minutes. Be sure to flip over occasionally, and spoon some of the marinade over the top.

⊙ Place the broccoli rabe in a steamer over boiling water and cook for 5 minutes. Remove from the steamer and plunge into a bowl of ice water.

⊙ Add coconut oil to a skillet over medium heat (making sure the oil doesn't smoke), and cook the tempeh for about 3–4 minutes on each side, until it becomes well browned. Keep warm.

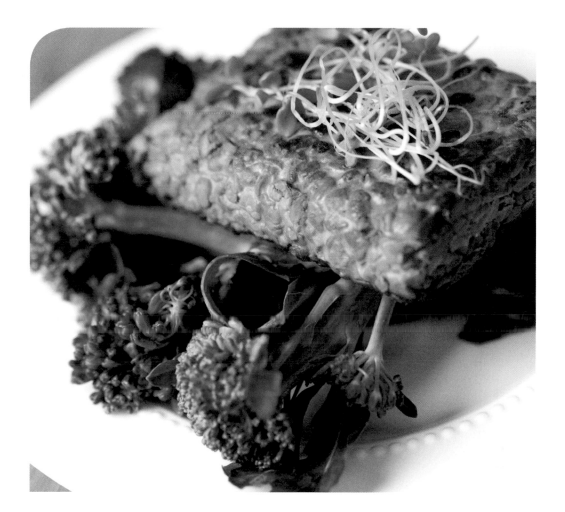

◉ Heat the vegetable broth in a skillet over medium-high heat, and sauté the garlic for a minute. Add the broccoli rabe and sauté for about 5 minutes, turning it from time to time. Do not overcook; otherwise, it will become limp.

◉ Divide the broccoli rabe among 4 plates and give each serving a splash of the fresh lemon juice. Make sure the stalks are arranged in a flat row. Season with sea salt and black pepper, if desired.

◉ Lay the tempeh over the broccoli rabe and serve immediately.

CREAMY CASHEW-FREE VEGGIE KORMA

YIELD: 4–6 SERVINGS

If you love creamy flavors, you're in for a real treat here. The problem with most creamy foods is that creaminess usually comes from . . . well . . . cream, or in the vegan world, from a huge amount of creamy nuts like cashews, which would be quite fattening. This is the result of my experiments without using either cream or cashews.

You'll see that the combination of the ingredients, and especially the cheesiness of the nutritional yeast and the thickening of arrowroot starch make this a creamy delight— sans dairy *or* nuts! It begs to be eaten over quinoa or brown rice, and I happily oblige.

INGREDIENTS

2 Tbs. + 3½ cups low-sodium vegetable broth, divided

1 medium-sized yellow onion, diced

1½ tsp. minced ginger

3 small cloves garlic, or 2 medium ones, minced

1¾ cups coconut milk

1 Tbs. tomato paste from a glass container

⅛ tsp. cayenne pepper, or to taste

1½ tsp. coriander

¼ tsp. turmeric

½ tsp. garam masala

1 tsp. curry powder

High-quality sea salt, to taste

Freshly ground black pepper, to taste

2 Tbs. arrowroot starch

2 medium sweet potatoes, cut into 2-inch chunks

1 medium cauliflower or about 7–8 cups medium florets

4 medium carrots or about 1½ cups, peeled and sliced into ½-inch slices

1 Tbs. nutritional yeast

2 Tbs. fresh lime juice

Cooked quinoa or brown rice

Chopped parsley for garnish

DIRECTIONS:

⦿ Heat 2 Tbs. vegetable broth in a large saucepan, and sauté the onion, ginger and garlic. Next, stir in the coconut milk, tomato paste and the rest of the vegetable broth; bring to a boil, and then reduce to a simmer. Add the cayenne pepper, coriander, turmeric, garam masala, curry, sea salt and black pepper. Stir well. Next, put a cup of this mixture into a bowl and whisk in the arrowroot starch, making sure that all lumps are removed. Add back to the main pot.

⦿ Allow the mixture to simmer down for 45 minutes, so it gets thick and creamy.

⦿ Meanwhile, heat water to a boil, and steam the sweet potatoes in a steamer until they soften, about 8–10 minutes or so. Remove sweet potatoes, then gently steam the cauliflower and carrots for about 5–7 minutes, or until they soften but retain their firmness.

⦿ After about 45 minutes, add the nutritional yeast, lime juice and veggies to the mixture, and stir them in over the simmering heat for about 5 minutes before serving.

⦿ Adjust seasonings, making it more spicy with cayenne, if you like. Serve over quinoa or brown rice and garnish the top of each dish with freshly chopped parsley.

LENTIL-MUSHROOM TARTS

YIELD: EIGHT 3¼-INCH TARTS

My mom is a pro at making these now. These are tasty additions to top a salad or to eat on their own with a side of cooked veggies, such as grilled asparagus or sautéed spinach. You can also stuff them into collard greens and make another version of a Gorilla Wrap.

INGREDIENTS

2 Tbs. + 2¼ cups low-sodium vegetable broth

½ cup diced yellow onion

1 clove garlic, minced

2 cups (8 ounces) chopped Baby Bella mushrooms

1 tsp. dried thyme

½ tsp. dried oregano

¼ tsp. dried sage

½ cup green lentils, soaked and rinsed well

1 Tbs. Ener-G egg replacer, mixed with 4 Tbs. very hot water

1 cup Gluten-Free Bread Crumbs (see page 216)

High-quality sea salt, to taste

Freshly ground black pepper, to taste

Coconut oil, for greasing tartlet or brioche molds

DIRECTIONS:

⊙ Preprep: Soak lentils overnight in water and rinse well.

⊙ Heat 2 Tbs. vegetable broth in a large saucepan and cook the onion for 3–4 minutes. Add the garlic, mushrooms, thyme, oregano and sage and sauté for another few minutes, until the mushrooms have given up their juices and soften.

⊙ Stir in the green lentils and add the rest of the vegetable broth. Bring to a boil, then reduce the heat and simmer for about 25 minutes, or until the lentils are cooked through. Stir in the egg replacer/water combination. Spoon the mixture into a bowl and place in the fridge for about 45 minutes–1 hour to cool.

⊙ Close to the end of this time period, preheat the oven to 350°F, and grease a large baking sheet with coconut oil or use a Silpat or parchment paper to line the sheet.

⊙ Remove the mixture from the fridge, stir in the bread crumbs. Add sea salt and black pepper and adjust seasonings, to taste. Then press the mixture into mini round tartlet or mini brioche molds, which you can get at a kitchen store, greased with coconut oil.

⊙ Place on the baking sheet and bake for 20–25 minutes, or until they are firm. Allow to cool, then carefully flip over and remove from the molds before serving.

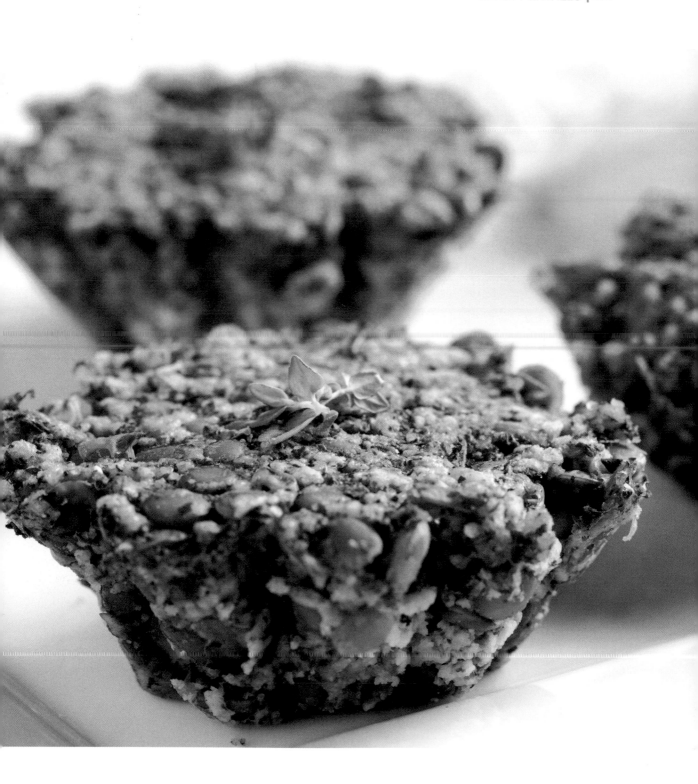

ALL-GREEN AND TEMPEH CALCIUM STIR-FRY

YIELD: 2 SERVINGS

Bok choy and sesame seeds are two of the best plant-based sources of calcium, making this dish an easy way to boost this beauty mineral in your diet.

INGREDIENTS

8 ounces tempeh

1 Tbs. coconut oil

1 Tbs. low-sodium vegetable broth

1 cup sliced white onions

1 garlic clove, minced

2 Tbs. low-sodium tamari

1 cup zucchini, cut into ½-inch slivers and then quarters

2 cups chopped bok choy, ends and much of the white stems trimmed off

1 cup asparagus tips and some of the green part of the stalk

2 tsp. sesame oil

1 tsp. raw apple cider vinegar

Pinch red pepper flakes

2 Tbs. sesame seeds

Microgreens, if desired

DIRECTIONS:

⊙ Bring a pot of water to a boil, then reduce heat and add tempeh. Simmer for 45 minutes. Once cooled, cut the tempeh into 1-inch pieces.

⊙ Heat the coconut oil in a large pan, and sauté the tempeh for a few minutes, until it starts to brown. Set to the side.

⊙ In the same pan, heat the vegetable broth, and begin to cook the onions over medium heat until translucent. Add the garlic, and cook for another minute.

⊙ Next add the tempeh and tamari, and gently stir, avoiding overly breaking up the tempeh. Make sure the tamari saturates the tempeh.

⊙ Add the zucchini, bok choy and asparagus, and cook for a few minutes, so they remain firm and don't get overcooked. Turn off the heat and add the sesame oil, raw apple cider vinegar and red pepper flakes, and stir.

⊙ Place the stir-fry on two plates and then top each with 1 Tbs. of sesame seeds and microgreens, if desired.

CRACKED CARAWAY SEED, BRUSSELS SPROUT, SQUASH AND CARROT STEW OVER BROWN RICE

YIELD: 2–3 SERVINGS

Orange is an auspicious color that many yogis and monks wear, and it is an abundant color in this dish. Here it indicates a wealth of beta-carotene (vitamin A), which is a powerful nutrient for beautiful skin and healthy hair. This dish is also an excellent way to enjoy the abundance of amino acids and calcium in Brussels sprouts.

DIRECTIONS:

⊙ Heat 1 Tbs. vegetable broth in a large saucepan, and sauté the shallots until translucent. Add the garlic, caraway seeds and thyme and sauté for another minute.

⊙ Add the Brussels sprouts, butternut squash and carrots, and stir for about 5 minutes. Next, add the rest of the vegetable broth. Raise the heat and bring to a boil, then reduce the heat to a simmer. Stir in the arrowroot starch, stirring constantly to remove any lumps. Simmer for about 40 minutes, or until the vegetables are cooked through and the liquid is reduced and thickened. Season with sea salt and black pepper, to suit your taste.

⊙ Serve over brown rice or quinoa.

INGREDIENTS

1 Tbs. + 4 cups low-sodium vegetable broth

3 Tbs. minced shallots

2 garlic cloves, minced

1 Tbs. caraway seeds

1 tsp. fresh thyme leaves, or ¼ tsp. dried thyme

4 cups Brussels sprouts, trimmed and halved

3½ cups peeled butternut squash, cubed into 1½-inch pieces

2 cups carrots, cut into 1-inch pieces on a bias

2 Tbs. arrowroot starch

High-quality sea salt, to taste

Freshly ground black pepper, to taste

Cooked brown rice or quinoa

SPINACH-BASIL POLENTA WITH CREAMY SAUCE

YIELD: 8–9 SERVINGS

BASE INGREDIENTS

6 cups spring or filtered water

2 cups finely ground polenta (choose organic polenta made with non-GMO corn)

3 Tbs. vegetable broth

2 cups coarsely chopped baby spinach

4 Tbs. nutritional yeast

3 Tbs. finely chopped fresh basil

High-quality sea salt, to taste

Freshly ground black pepper, to taste

Coconut oil, for greasing pan

SAUCE INGREDIENTS

2½ cups coconut milk

2 Tbs. minced baby spinach

1 Tbs. minced basil

½ tsp. xanthan gum

High-quality sea salt, to taste

Freshly ground black pepper, to taste

To make a creamy vegan dish, many recipes call for vegan butter spreads. These are full of polyunsaturated oils or a heavy cashew base, neither of which I recommend using. This dish doesn't include oils or a cashew base. Instead, coconut milk lends a satisfying, creamy texture to this dish. Serve with greens, such as arugula, which will add a spicy bite to the creamy texture of the polenta.

I don't eat a lot of corn, since it is not as nutrient-dense as many other veggies and is often genetically modified, but I do like this polenta version, made with organic, non-GMO corn.

DIRECTIONS:

◉ In a large pot, bring water to a boil. Reduce heat and stir in the polenta, stirring constantly. Keep stirring and stirring!

◉ Meanwhile, heat the vegetable broth and quickly sauté the spinach, just until it wilts, and set it to the side. Keep stirring the polenta for a total of about 45 minutes, or until it becomes too thick to stir, then stir in the spinach at the last moment.

◉ Turn off the heat and add the nutritional yeast and basil. Add the sea salt and black pepper, to taste.

◉ Grease a 9 x 9 inch Pyrex baking pan with coconut oil. Add the mixture to the pan and press down with the back of a spoon. Let it sit for about 20 minutes or so to set. You can keep it warm in the oven at the "warming" or lowest temperature setting.

RAW CORAZON CHILI

YIELD: 3–4 SERVINGS

This raw chili dish bears a strong resemblance to the consistency, texture and flavor of meat-based chili. I was forced to invent it for a client who seriously missed chili after completely giving up red meat. If you warm it up a bit, as I suggest, it will be a satisfying dish in the winter. Pair with a green salad, per our usual Beauty Detox meal-ordered protocol.

DIRECTIONS:

◉ Put the carrots in a large bowl.

◉ Add the portobello mushroom, sun-dried tomatoes, almonds, spices, lime juice, olive oil and water to the work bowl of a food processor with the blade in place. Process to a chunky consistency. Be careful not to make the mixture too smooth.

◉ Add the processed mixture to the bowl with the carrots and stir to combine well. You can warm the chili gently in a large pot or in the bottom of the dehydrator about half an hour before serving. Serve in warm bowls, garnished with cilantro.

INGREDIENTS

1½ cups peeled and chopped carrots

1 large portobello mushroom cap

1½ cups sun-dried tomatoes (soaked for 2 hours in warm water if totally dry and hard)

1 cup almonds, soaked overnight and rinsed well

⅓ tsp. high-quality sea salt

2 Tbs. chili powder

1 Tbs. cumin

½ Tbs. paprika

1½ Tbs. fresh lime juice

2 tsp. olive oil

1½ cups cold filtered water

Cilantro, for garnish

RAW NO-BEAN REFRIED BEANS

YIELD: ABOUT 2½ CUPS

INGREDIENTS

2 cups sunflower seeds, soaked overnight and rinsed well

1 cup sun-dried tomatoes (soaked in a bowl for 2 hours prior to blending)

2 Tbs. freshly ground flaxseeds

1 Tbs. raw unpasteurized miso paste

½ Tbs. paprika

2 tsp. chili powder

¼ tsp. cayenne pepper

¼–½ cup spring or filtered water (depending on the consistency of your sun-dried tomatoes)

High-quality sea salt, to taste

Sun-dried tomatoes, when processed together with sunflower seeds, mimic that beanlike consistency you may know and love. This dish is great on salads or in wraps. Unlike overcooked beans, sunflower seeds help produce that inner glow (see Chapter 8). I make sure to eat some every week.

DIRECTIONS:

⊙ Pulse the sunflower seeds in the food processor, and then add the sun-dried tomatoes, flaxseeds, miso paste and seasonings. Pulse again, then slowly add the water to the mixture until it has a consistency that resembles refried beans—almost smooth, but with some texture. Mix in some sea salt to suit your taste.

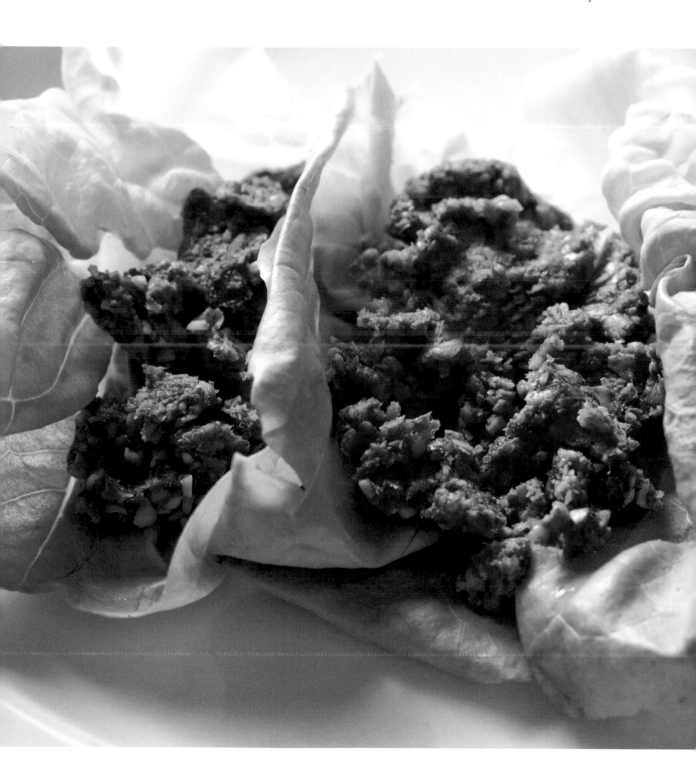

RAW CURRIED INDIAN VEGGIES

YIELD: 6–8 SERVINGS

INGREDIENTS

2 red peppers, cored and sliced into ¼-inch strips

1 medium head cauliflower, cut into florets

½ medium white onion, sliced thinly

¼ cup cold, filtered water

1 Tbs. coconut oil

2 tsp. curry

¼ tsp. turmeric

¼ tsp. paprika

¾ tsp. high-quality sea salt

½ cup sunflower seeds, soaked overnight and rinsed thoroughly

½ cup pumpkin seeds, soaked overnight and rinsed thoroughly

Ever since spending three months in India, I am a huge India-phile. I love all things Indian, including the culture, people, clothing, bright colors of the temples and decor, yoga, meditation practices that focus on seeking happiness from within, spices and, yes, Indian food. However, I don't love how much veggies can sometimes be overcooked, or how cream and clarified butter are often slipped into some veg-etarian dishes. I love this dish for bringing out the flavors in Indian food—the curry and turmeric—in a totally healthful and beautifying way. *Om Shanti!*

DIRECTIONS:

⊙ Place the red peppers, cauliflower and onion in a large bowl and set aside.

⊙ Place the rest of the ingredients, except for the seeds, in the work bowl of a food processor with the blade in place, and process until thoroughly combined. Add the seeds and process until the mixture is thick and chunky.

⊙ Spoon the mixture over the veggies in the bowl, and mix very well with your hands. Because the mixture will be a thick paste, I find that using your hands is the best way to saturate all the veggies evenly with the mixture.

⊙ Spread over Teflex sheets in the dehydrator and dehydrate for 5–6 hours at 110°F, or until the vegetables are softened and warmed. If you don't have a dehydrator, spread the mixture on baking sheets and bake in the oven, at the lowest temperature with the door cracked open, for about 2 hours.

RAW PAD THAI

YIELD: 3–4 SERVINGS

Thailand is one of the countries closest to my heart. It was the place where I landed after leaving Australia during my around-the-world journey, and it welcomed me warmly. When I look back on the months I spent there, island hopping, living with hill tribes in the north and exploring dozens of Buddhist temples, I recall amazing memories of times I spent in Bangkok, meeting other backpackers while staying on the Koh San Road.

On Koh San, there are dozens of street vendors. For 15 baht (at the time, around 50 cents), I would buy a little container of pad thai. That was great for me, as I was on a strict backpacker's budget. The vendor knew how I liked it: mostly veggie, very little oil and no egg. This version of pad thai helps take me back there.

Kelp noodles are an amazingly nutritious alternative to grain-based noodles, with virtually no calories (6 calories for 4 ounces). They're sold at certain health food stores, but if you have trouble finding them, the Sea Tangle brand sells them online at a reasonable price by the case.

DIRECTIONS:

⦿ In a food processor or blender, process the dressing ingredients until smooth, adding the almond butter last. Set aside.

⦿ Rinse the kelp noodles thoroughly and drain in a colander. Add to a large bowl, and toss with the dressing, green onions and tomato.

⦿ Serve at room temperature or warm over low heat. Spoon into individual warm bowls. Garnish each bowl with chopped nuts and a wedge of lime.

DRESSING INGREDIENTS

2 Tbs. sesame seeds

2 Tbs. sesame oil

3 Tbs. rice vinegar

¼ tsp. red pepper flakes

⅓ cup sun-dried tomatoes (soaked in a bowl for 2 hours prior to blending)

2 Tbs. coconut nectar or maple syrup

1 tsp. powdered stevia

2 Tbs. low-sodium tamari

2 Tbs. lime juice

2 Tbs. raw almond butter

BASE INGREDIENTS

2 packages kelp noodles, or about 24 ounces

1 cup chopped green onions, white part only

1 medium slicing tomato, cut into 1-inch cubes

1 cup finely chopped macadamia or pine nuts, as a garnish

1 lime, cut into quarters, as a garnish

RAW ZUCCHINI PESTO PASTA

YIELD: 2–3 SERVINGS

INGREDIENTS

2–3 medium zucchinis (depending on size), peeled and cut into curly noodles with a spiralizer

Raw, Lighter Pesto Dressing (see page 190)

You can find a fairly inexpensive spiralizer online or at your local cooking shop. Mine was around $30. It's super fun to make pastalike shapes with vegetables, which absorb sauce really well. The key is to let the zucchini "noodles" sit out for a while to warm to room temperature. I find cold raw food very unappealing. With the delicious pesto dressing, this is a great dish.

DIRECTIONS:

⦿ Spiralize the zucchini and place it in a bowl.

⦿ Top with a generous portion of dressing, and toss well.

NOTE: It's best to leave the spiralized zucchini out at room temperature for about 3 hours before serving. It will soften a bit and become more like real pasta. Serve at room temperature, or warmed for 30 minutes in the dehydrator or the oven at the lowest temperature, with the door cracked open.

RAW FALAFEL

YIELD: ABOUT 7 FALAFEL BALLS

This is a raw version of a dish that's usually fried. I love it on salad or to make collard green wraps. Be sure to start soaking the necessary nuts and seeds the night before you plan to serve it.

DIRECTIONS:

⊙ In the work bowl of a food processor with the blade in place, pulse all the seeds and nuts, keeping the texture chunky. Add the rest of the ingredients, except dressing, and pulse again until the mixture is moist.

⊙ Wet your hands slightly, and form with your hands into balls slightly smaller than Ping-Pong balls.

⊙ Warm them gently in your oven at the lowest setting with the door cracked open for an hour or more (monitor for the warmth you prefer), or dehydrate for $3\frac{1}{2}$ hours at 110°F, and serve warm right out of the dehydrator, topped with dressing.

INGREDIENTS

½ cup almonds, soaked overnight and rinsed well

½ cup walnuts, soaked 2 hours

2 Tbs. sesame seeds, ideally soaked overnight

2 Tbs. sunflower seeds, soaked overnight

1½ Tbs. olive oil

¼ tsp. freshly ground black pepper

1 very small or ½ a medium clove garlic, minced

2 Tbs. finely chopped white onion

½ tsp. high-quality sea salt

½ Tbs. minced fresh sage

½ Tbs. fresh thyme leaves

2½ Tbs. packed minced parsley

Creamy Dijon-Tahini Dressing (see page 190)

RAW ASIAN CREAMY KELP NOODLES

YIELD: 3–4 SERVINGS

Kelp noodles contain virtually no calories (6 calories for 4 ounces), yet are very high in minerals. I give them to my clients often as a substitute for other types of noodles or pastas, especially when they are trying to lose weight.

The scallions, tomato and purple cabbage add vibrant color, vitamins and minerals.

If you are after a really creamy texture, this one's for you. This is one of the few recipes where I've included cashews. Remember they should be eaten in moderation and not very often. Cashews are almost always steamed out of their shell, so you will rarely, if ever, encounter truly raw cashews. Still, enjoy them in this dish, as an occasional treat.

Be sure to store all nuts in the fridge to prevent them from becoming rancid.

INGREDIENTS

2 packages raw kelp noodles, 24 ounces

¼ cup water

1 Tbs. miso paste

1½ Tbs. sesame oil

1½ cups + ⅓ cup unroasted cashews, divided

½ tsp. high-quality sea salt

1 cup chopped scallions, white part only

1¼ cups diced tomato

1¼ cups sliced red cabbage

Fresh cilantro, for garnish

1 lime, quartered, for garnish

DIRECTIONS:

⊙ Rinse the kelp noodles well in a colander. Place in a large mixing bowl and set aside.

⊙ In a blender, process the water, miso paste, sesame oil, 1½ cups of the raw cashews, and sea salt until thoroughly combined. Pour over the kelp noodles and mix well. This is best done with clean hands, which helps to evenly saturate the noodles with the sauce.

⊙ Add the raw veggies. Mix well again with your hands, and divide equally among 4 plates. Grind the last ⅓ cup of cashews in a food processor. Garnish each dish with a sprig of cilantro, a sprinkling of ground cashews and a quarter of a lime.

⊙ Serve at room temperature or warm very gently in a pot.

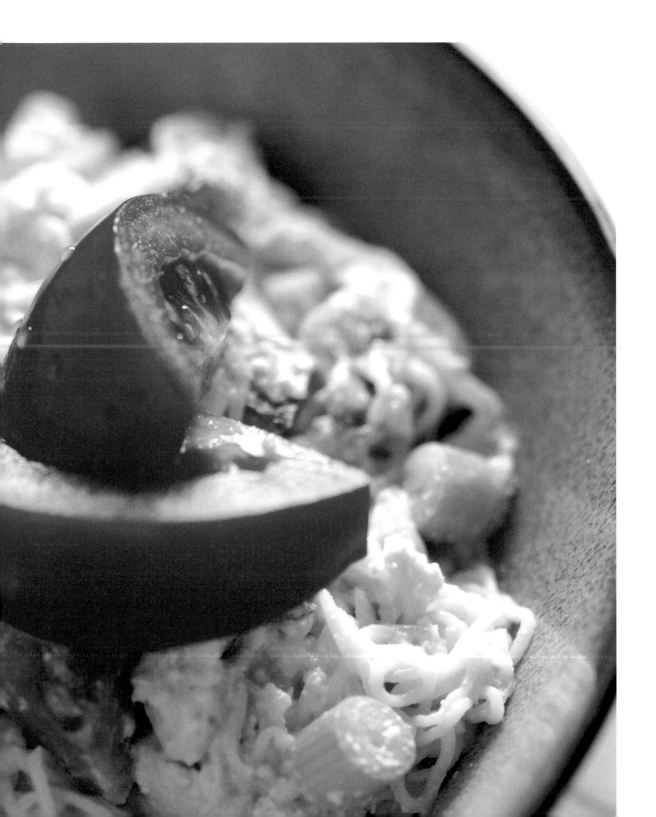

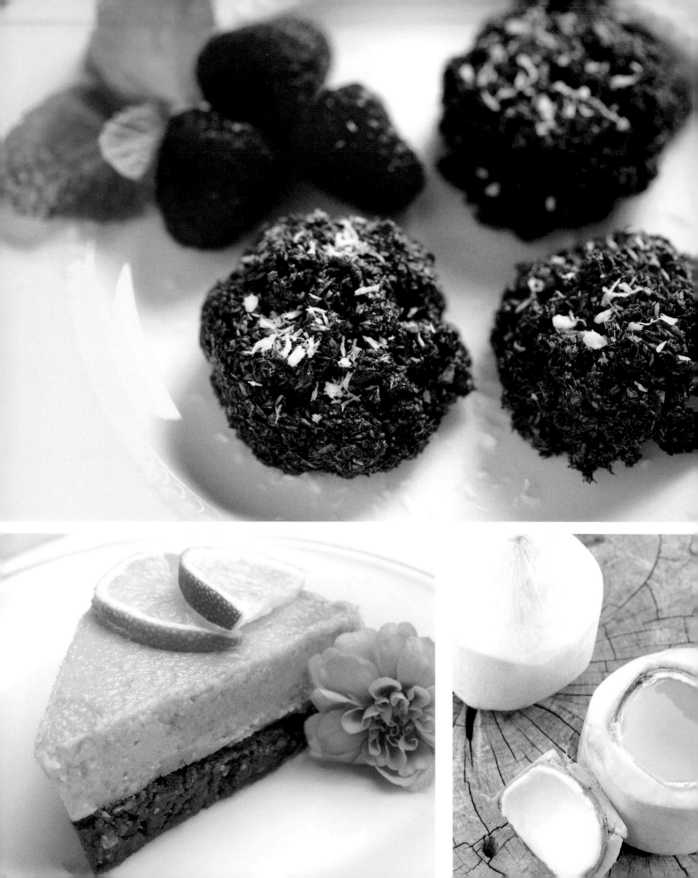

BEAUTY DESSERTS

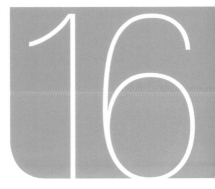

RAW CHOCOLATE GINGER STACKED CAKE WITH FROSTING

YIELD: 6 PIECES

CAKE INGREDIENTS

1 cup almonds

¾ cup walnuts

¼ cup raw cacao

¼ tsp. high-quality sea salt

1 tsp. grated ginger

3 Tbs. raw coconut nectar (or maple syrup)

5 Medjool dates, pitted

1 tsp. vanilla

FROSTING INGREDIENTS

¾ cup avocado flesh

3 dates

2 Tbs. cacao powder

¼ cup raw coconut nectar

Fresh mint, as a garnish (optional)

This is a sexy recipe that you can make for your significant other or for your friends, before a fun night out . . . or in! Dark chocolate has a centuries-old reputation as an aphrodisiac and contains the compound phenylethylamine, or PEA, which creates an emotional high similar to being in love. Serotonin is another chemical known to be released in your brain when you're eating chocolate, which fosters a sense of well-being.

Ginger spices things up and increases circulation and body temperature.

Avocado gives the frosting its silky smoothness, without the use of cream or dairy products. This sexy fruit has a reputation as an aphrodisiac extending back to ancient Aztec times. In fact, the Aztecs called the avocado tree *Ahuacuatl,* which translates to "testicle tree." I kid you not.

When you want an occasional chocolate treat, this is a healthier way to get your fix!

DIRECTIONS:

⊙ Process the almonds, walnuts and cacao in a food processor and grind well. Add the sea salt, ginger, coconut nectar, dates and vanilla and mix again until a smooth mixture is formed.

⊙ Press the mixture firmly into an 8 x 6 inch rectangular glass baking dish, or a dish of a similar size. Cut in half and separate with a spatula, as you will be stacking one half of the cake on top of the other.

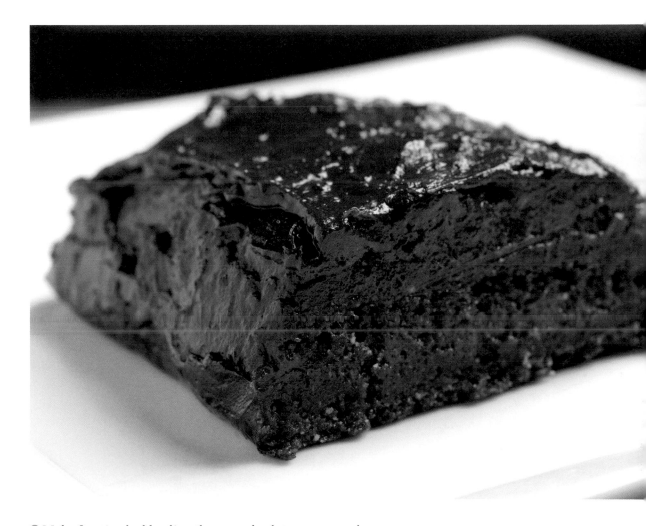

⊙ Make frosting by blending the avocado, dates, cacao and coconut nectar in a blender or food processor. Use half the frosting to frost one of the halves, then stack the other half of the cake carefully on top. Finally, frost the top of the double-layered cake with the remainder of the frosting.

⊙ Slice into pieces lengthwise and across. Garnish with a little mint on the side to add a pop of color.

FRESH PR COCONUT MEAT YOGURT AND COCONUT WATER KEFIR

YIELD: ABOUT ²/₃ CUP AND 1 QUART

INGREDIENTS

5 young coconuts

¾ tsp. + 1 tsp. kefir starter culture, divided

I included *PR* in the name of this recipe as a nod to Puerto Rico, which I love dearly and where I eat coconuts almost constantly whenever I visit. The young coconuts you'll find to make this fresh yogurt and kefir may not be right off the tree, but those coconuts are divine as well.

Making your own fresh coconut yogurt offers the advantage of yogurt with no additives or preservatives of any kind. The potent tanginess and freshness can't be beat. It may be more realistic for your lifestyle to buy coconut yogurt, which is widely available now in health food markets, but when you have the chance to make it, you will love the result. You're also getting a two for one bonus in this recipe, as we are using the coconut meat to make the yogurt and the coconut water to make the kefir.

DIRECTIONS:

FRESH PR COCONUT MEAT YOGURT

⊙ Crack open the young coconuts using a cleaver and scrape out the meat, rinsing off any small wood pieces and adding to the blender or food processor. Check out my demo video on how to safely open young coconuts on www.kimberlysnyder. net if you are a newbie. Pour the coconut water into a sterilized jar. Blend the meat until smooth and add to a sterilized bowl.

⊙ Mix in ¾ tsp. of the live starter kefir culture. You can buy this at a health food store or online. Though the kefir starter may have been cultured in dairy, and say that on the label, very little actual dairy should be left in the kefir starter. Cover the bowl with a paper towel or cheesecloth and seal with a rubber band. Leave in a warm place (ideally at least around 70°F). Check the yogurt after 8–12 hours. It should have a tangy flavor, and be a bit thicker. If it isn't that tangy yet, leave it for another 4–8 hours, checking up on it for that tangy yogurt taste. The longer you leave it, the more sour it will turn, so if you prefer your yogurt more sour than sweet, leave it on the longer side.

⊙ Once you deem it ready, you can move it into the fridge, where it will keep for a few weeks but will start to sour more over time.

FRESH PR COCONUT WATER KEFIR

⊙ Next, take the coconut water and heat in a pot on low, until it rooms to warm temperature. Whatever you do, don't boil the water! When the water is warm (about 92°F), whisk in 1 tsp. of the starter kefir culture. Pour into a sterilized jar or a container and keep out at room temperature, covered, for 24 hours. Move into the fridge, and start consuming one ounce at a time, building up from there. It too should taste tangy. It can be consumed at any time during the day.

⊙ Use some of this batch as the starter for your next batch (for a quart, use 6 Tbs.) within two or three days of fermenting the first batch, and you'll never have to buy a starter again

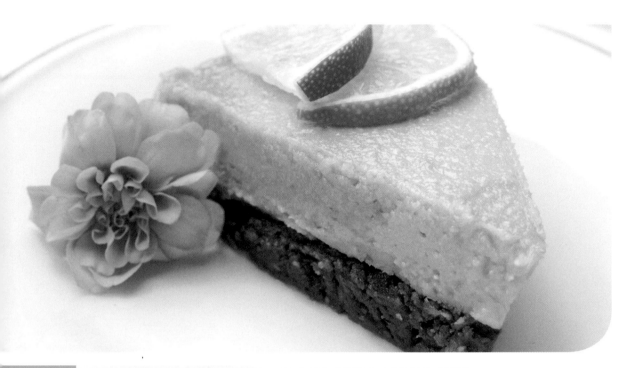

CRUST INGREDIENTS

1 cup raw walnuts, soaked for 15 minutes and rinsed well

¾ cup raw pecans

4 dates, pitted

2½ Tbs. raw coconut nectar or maple syrup

¼ tsp. high-quality sea salt

FILLING INGREDIENTS

¾ cup fresh lime juice

2 cups raw cashews

½ cup raw coconut nectar or maple syrup

⅓ cup coconut oil

¾ tsp. vanilla extract

RAW KEY LIME PIE

YIELD: ONE 9-INCH PIE

This is a great lime-lover's dessert. It does contain cashews, so enjoy in moderation.

DIRECTIONS:

⊙ Put all the crust ingredients together in the work bowl of a food processor with the blade in place and process until the ingredients form a ball. Press into a 9-inch Pyrex pie pan.

⊙ Wash and dry the food processor bowl and blade. Add the filling ingredients to the bowl with the blade in place. Blend the filling ingredients together in the processor, and pour over the crust. Place in the freezer and allow to set for at least 3 hours or overnight. Take it out and let it rest at room temperature for about 10 minutes, or as long as it takes to soften, before serving.

CONVERTING TO METRIC

VOLUME MEASUREMENT CONVERSIONS

U.S.	METRIC
¼ teaspoon	1.25 ml
½ teaspoon	2.5 ml
¾ teaspoon	3.75 ml
1 teaspoon	5 ml
1 tablespoon	15 ml
¼ cup	62.5 ml
½ cup	125 ml
¾ cup	187.5 ml
1 cup	250 ml

WEIGHT MEASUREMENT CONVERSIONS

U.S.	METRIC
1 ounce	28.4 g
8 ounces	227.5 g
16 ounces (1 pound)	455 g

COOKING TEMPERATURE CONVERSIONS

Celsius/Centigrade	0°C and 100°C are the freezing and boiling points of water, respectively, and are standard to the metric system.
Fahrenheit	Fahrenheit established 0°F as the stabilized temperature when equal amounts of ice, water and salt are mixed. Water freezes at 32°F and boils at 212°F.

To convert temperatures in Fahrenheit to Celsius, use this formula:
C = (F – 32) x 0.5555

So, for example, if you are baking at 350°F and want to know that temperature in Celsius, your calculation would be:
C = (350 – 32) x 0.5555 = 176.65°C

ENDNOTES

CHAPTER ONE

1. Tom Bohager, *Enzymes: What the Experts Know* (Prescott, AZ: One World Press, 2006), 40.

2. Some of this information was paraphrased from these books: Viktoras Kulvinskas, *Survival in the 21st Century* (Wethersfield, CT: Omangod Press, 1979), 193; Adina Niemerow, *Super Cleanse* (New York: HarperCollins, 2008), 70.

3. Robert Young, Ph.D., *The pH Miracle* (New York: Wellness Central, Hachette Book Group, 2002), 42.

4. Norman W. Walker, *Colon Health* (Prescott, AZ: Norwalk Press, 1979), 3.

5. Gene Stone, ed. *Forks Over Knives: The Plant-Based Way to Health* (New York: The Experiment, LLC, 2011), 5, 10.

6. John Scharffenberg, *Problems with Meat* (Anaheim, CA: Woodbridge Press, 1982), 90; Nathan Prikitin, *Vegetarian Times* 43: 21.

7. Dr. Gary Farr, "Comparing Organic Versus Commercially Grown Foods," Rutgers University Study, New Brunswick, NJ, 2002.

8. Gabriel Cousens, M.D., *Rainbow Green Live-Food Cuisine* (Berkeley, CA: North Atlantic Books, 2003), 68–79.

9. Environmental Working Group (**www.ewg.org**), 2012.

10. E. C. Westman, W. S. Yancy, J. S. Edman, et al., "Carbohydrate Diet Program," *American Journal of Medicine* 113 (2002): 30–36.

11. R. C. Atkins, *Dr. Atkins' New Diet Revolution* (New York: Avon Books, 1999).

12. Westman, Yancy, Edman, et al., "Carbohydrate Diet Program."

13. John A. McDougall, M.D., *The McDougall Program for Maximum Weight Loss* (New York: Penguin, 1995), 46.

14. Gabriel Cousens, M.D., *Conscious Eating* (Berkeley, CA: North Atlantic Books, 2000), 313.

15. Richard J. Johnson, M.D., *The Sugar Fix: The High-Fructose Fallout That Is Making You Fat and Sick* (New York: Rodale, 2008), 118.

16. S. A. Bilsborough and T. C. Crowe, "Low-Carbohydrate Diets: What Are the Potential Short- and Long-Term Health Implications?" *Asia Pacific Journal of Clinical Nutrition* 13 (2003): 396–404.

17. C. Paul Bianchi and Russell Hilf, *Protein Metabolism and Biological Function* (New Brunswick, NJ: Rutgers University Press, 1970).

18. Statement by Margaret Mellon, Ph.D., J.D., director of the UCS Food and Environment Program and coauthor of the Union of Concerned Scientists report "Hogging It: Estimates of Antimicrobial Abuse in Livestock," given at the press conference announcing the report's release, January 8, 2001. **www.ucsusa.org/**

19. Emily Oken, M.D., K. P. Kleinman, W. E. Berland et al., "Decline in Fish Consumption Among Pregnant Women after a National Mercury Advisory," *Obstetrics and Gynecology* 102 (2003): 346–351. **www.greejournal.org/cgi/content/full/102/2/346**

20. Lynn R. Goldman, M.D., M.P.H. and M. W. Shannon, "American Academy of Pediatrics: Technical Report: Mercury in the Environment: Implications for Pediatricians," *Pediatrics* 108, no. 1 (2001): 197–205.

21. U.S. Food and Drug Administration, "What You Need to Know About Mercury in Fish and Shellfish." **www.fda.gov/food/foodsafety/product-specificinformation/seafood/foodbornepathogenscontaminants/methylmercury/ucm115644.htm**

22. Natural Resources Defense Council, "Mercury Contamination in Fish." **www.nrdc.org/health/effects/mercury/guide.asp**

23. Interview with Dr. Neal Barnard, author of *Foods That Fight Pain.* "Go Vegetarian, Go Vegan! Starter Kit. Eating for Life," PETA, 4 (February 15, 2011).

24. Elson M. Haas, M.D. with Buck Levin, Ph.D., R.D., *Staying Healthy with Nutrition: The Complete Guide to Diet and Nutritional Medicine* (Berkeley, CA: Celestial Arts, 2006), 558.

25. Dr. T. Colin Campbell and Thomas M Campbell II, *The China Study: The Most Comprehensive Study of Nutrition Ever Conducted and the Startling Implications for Diet, Weight Loss, and Long-Term Health* (Dallas: Benbella Books, 2006), 6.

26. Campbell and Campbell, *The China Study,* 6.

27. Harvey Diamond and Marilyn Diamond, *Fit for Life* (New York: Warner Books, 1985), 107.

28. K. L. Reichelt, A.-M. Knivsberg, G. Lind and M. Nødland, "Probable Etiology and Possible Treatment of Childhood Autism," *Brain Dysfunction* 4 (1991): 308–319.

29. J. M. Ohan and E. L. Giovannucci, "Dairy Products, Calcium, and Vitamin D and Risk of Prostate Cancer," *Epidemiological Reviews* 23 (2001), 87–92.

30. http://en.wikipedia.org/wiki/Hiromi Shinya

31. Hiromi Shinya, M.D., *The Enzyme Factor* (Tulsa, OK: Council Oak Books, 2007).

32. Young, *The pH Miracle,* 45.

33. Dr. Joel Fuhrman, *Eat to Live* (New York: Little, Brown and Company, 2003), 84.

34. S. Maggi, J. L. Kelsey, J. Litvak and S. P. Hayes, "Incidence of Hip Fractures in the Elderly: A Cross-National Analysis." *Osteoporosis International* 1, no. 4 (1991): 232–241.

35. B. J. Abelow, T. R. Holford and K. L. Insogna, "Cross-Cultural Association between Dietary Animal Protein and Hip Fracture: A Hypothesis," *Calcified Tissue International* 50 (1992): 14–18.

36. Cited in Furhman, *Eat to Live,* 85.

CHAPTER TWO

1. Humbart Santillo, *Food Enzymes: The Missing Link to Radiant Health* (Prescott, AZ: Hohm Press, 1993).

2. Tom Bohager, *Enzymes: What the Experts Know* (Prescott, AZ: One World Press, 2006), 55.

3. Young, *The pH Miracle,* 5–6, 15.

4. Jane E. Brody, "Exploring a Low-Acid Diet for Bone Health," *New York Times,* (November 23, 2009): www.nytimes.com/2009/11/24/health/24brod.html?_r=0

5. Ibid.

6. Daniel DeNoon, "Drink More Diet Soda, Gain More Weight?" *Web MD Medical News* (June 13, 2005). www.webmd.com/content/Article/107/108476.htm

7. G. R. Howe, "Dietary Intake of Fiber and Decreased Risk of Cancers of the Colon and the Rectum: Evidence from the Combined Analysis of 13 Case-Control Studies," *Journal of the National Cancer Institute* 84, no. 24 (December 1992): 1887–1896.

8. John A. McDougall, *Digestive Tune-Up* (Summertown, TN: Healthy Living Publications, 2008), 76.

9. Ibid.

10. Dr. Mercola, "Can Low Doses of Allergens Cure the Allergies Themselves?" (June 27, 2009). www.mercola.com

11. James Braly, M.D. and Ron Hoggan, M.A., *Dangerous Grains: Why Gluten Cereal Grains May Be Hazardous to Your Health* (New York: Avery, 2002).

12. M. Lenoir, F. Serre, L. Cantin, S. H. Ahmed (2007). "Intense Sweetness Surpasses Cocaine Reward," *PloS ONE* 2, no. 8 (2007): e698.

13. H. A. Jamel and J. Dent, "Taste Preference for Sweetness in Urban and Rural Populations in Iraq," *Journal of Dental Research* 75, no. 11 (November 1996): 1879–1884.

14. A. T. Lee and A. Cerami, "The Role of Glycation in Aging," *Annals of the New York Academy of Science* 663, (1992): 63–70.

15. D. G. Dyer et al., "Accumulation of Maillard Reaction Products in Skin Collagen in Diabetes and Aging," *Journal of Clinical Investigation* 93, no. 6 (1993): 421–422.

16. F. Couzy, C. Keen, M. E. Gershwin et al., "Nutritional Implications of the Interactions Between Minerals," *Progressive Food and Nutrition Science* 17 (1933): 65–87; A. Kozlovsky, P. B. Moser, S. Reiser, et al., "Effects of Diets High in Simple Sugars on Urinary Chromium Losses," *Metabolism* 35, (June 1986): 515–518; M. Fields, R. J. Ferretti, J. C. Smith Jr, et al., "Effect of Copper Deficiency on Metabolism and Mortality in Rats Fed Sucrose or Starch Diets," *Journal of Clinical Nutrition* 113 (1983): 1335–1345; J. Lemann, "Evidence that Glucose Ingestion Inhibits Net Renal Tubular Reabsorption of Calcium and Magnesium," *Journal of Clinical Nutrition* 70 (1976): 236–245.

17. P. Mohanty, W. Hamouda, R. Garg, et al. "Glucose Challenge Stimulates Reactive Oxygen Species (ROS) Generation by Leucocytes," *Journal of Clinical Endocrinology and Metabolism* 85, no. 8 (August 2000): 2970–2973.

18. Nancy Appleton, *Lick the Sugar Habit* (New York: Avery Penguin Putnam, 1988).

19. F. Lechin, B. van der Dijs, M. Lechin, et al., "Effects of an Oral Glucose Load on Plasma Neurotransmitters in Humans," *Neuropsychobiology* 265, nos. 1–2 (1992): 4–11.

20. F. S. Goulart, "Are You Sugar Smart?" *American Fitness* (March–April 1991): 34–38.

21. Family Education.com, "Healthy Habits: Cut Back on Refined Sugars," excerpted from David and Anne Frahm, *Healthy Habits: 20 Simple Ways to Improve Your Health* (New York: Penguin Putnam Inc., 2003.)

22. Johnson, *The Sugar Fix*, 123.

23. M. Chandalia, A. Garg, D. Lutjoham, et al., "Beneficial Effects of High Dietary Fiber Intake in Patients with Type-2 Diabetes Mellitus," *New England Journal of Medicine* 342, no. 19 (2000): 1392–1398.

24. Johnson, *The Sugar Fix*, 199.

25. Elizabeth J. Parks, Lauren E. Skokan, Maureen T. Timlin and Carlus S. Dingfelder, "Dietary Sugars Stimulate Fatty Acid Synthesis in Adults," *Journal of Nutrition* 138 (June 2008): 1039–1046.

26. Miriam E. Bocarsly, Elyse S. Powell, Nicole M. Avena and Bartley G. Hoebel, "High-Fructose Corn Syrup Causes Characteristic of Obesity in Rats: Increased Body Weight, Body Fat and Triglyceride Levels," *Pharmacology Biochemistry and Behavior* (2010), DOI: 10.1016/j. pbb.2010.02.012.

27. Dr. Joseph Mercola, "Shocking! This 'Tequila' Sweetener is Far Worse than High Fructose Corn Syrup" (March 30, 2010). **www.mercola.com**

28. Roger B. McDonald, "Influence of Dietary Sucrose on Biological Aging," *American Journal of Clinical Nutrition* 62 (1995): 284S–293S.

29. Johnson, *The Sugar Fix,* 98.

30. John Kohler, "The Truth about Agave Syrup: Not as Healthy as You May Think." **www.living-foods.com**

31. W. L. Hall, D. J. Millward, P. J. Rogers and L. M. Morgan, "Physiological Mechanisms Mediating Aspartame-Induced Satiety," *Physiology & Behavior* 78, nos. 4–5 (April 2003): 557–562.

32. L. N. Chen and E. S. Parham, "College Students' Use of High-Intensity Sweeteners is Not Consistently Associated with Sugar Consumption," *Journal of the American Dietetic Association* 91 (1991): 686–690.

33. Susan E. Swithers and Terry L. Davidson, "A Role for Sweet Taste: Calorie Predictive Relations in Energy Regulation by Rats" *Behavioral Neuroscience* 122, no. 1 (February 2008): 161–173.

34. Mohamed B. Abou-Donia, Eman M. El-Masry, Ali A. Abdel-Rahman, et al., "Splenda Alters Gut Microflora and Increases Intestinal P-Glycoprotein and Cytochrome P-450 in Male Rats," *Journal of Toxicology and Environmental Health,* Part A 71, no. 21 (2008): 1415–1429.

35. Patti Weller, *The Power of Nutrient-Dense Food: How to Use Food to Feel Great, Lose Weight and Prevent Disease* (El Cajon, CA: Deerpath Publishing Company, 2005), 28.

36. Akihiro Okitani, Seung-Yed Kim, Fumitaka Hayase, et al., "Heat Induced Changes in Free Amino Acids on Manufactured Heated Pulps and Pastes from Tomatoes," *Journal of Food Science* 48 (1983): 1366–1367.

37. Cited in Dr. Gabriel Cousens, *Rainbow Green Live-Food Cuisine,* 56.

38. Winston J. Craig, Ph.D., M.P.H., R.D. and Ann Reed Mangels, Ph.D., R.D., L.D.N., F.A.D.A., "Position of the American Dietetic Association: Vegetarian Diets." *Journal of the American Dietetic Association* 109, no. 7 (2009): 1267–1268.

39. C. Adams, *Handbook of the Nutritional Value of Foods in Common Units* (New York: Dover Publications, 1986).

40. A. Costantini, Heinrich Wieland and Lars I. Qvick, *Etiology and Prevention of Atherosclerosis* (Freiburg, Germany: Ludwigs School of Medicine, 2002).

41. M. C. Lancaster, F. P. Jenkins and J. M. Philip, "Toxicity Associated with Certain Samples of Ground Nuts." *Nature* 192 (1961): 1095–1096.

42. G. N. Wogan and P. M. Newberne, "Dose-Response Characteristics of Aflatoxin B1 Carcinogenesis in the Rat," *Cancer Research* 27 (1967): 2370–2376; G. N. Wogan, S. Paglialunga and P. M. Newberne, "Carcinogenic Effects of Low Dietary Levels of Aflatoxin B1 in Rats," *Food and Cosmetics Toxicology* 12 (1974): 681–685.

43. Environment, Health and Safety online. **www.ehso.com/ehshome/aflatoxin.php**

44. Elson Haas, M.D., *Staying Healthy with Nutrition: The Complete Guide to Diet & Nutritional Medicine* (Berkeley, CA: Celestial Arts, 2006).

45. Sally Fallon and Mary G. Enig, Ph.D., "Newest Research on Why You Should Avoid Soy," *Nexus Magazine* 7, no. 3 (April–May 2000).

46. Cousens, *Rainbow Green Live-Food Cuisine,* 89.

47. Joseph J. Rackis, M. R. Gumbmann, I. E. Liener, "The USDA Trypsin Inhibitor Study. I. Background, Objectives and Procedural Details," *Qualification of Plant Foods in Human Nutrition* 35 (1985).

48. R. L. Divi, H. C. Chang and D. R. Doerge, "Identification, Characterization and Mechanisms of Anti-Thyroid Activity of Isoflavones from Soybeans," *Biochemical Pharmacology* 54 (1997): 1087–1096.

49. Daniel R. Doerge, "Inactivation of Thyroid Peroxidase by Genistein and Daidzein in Vitro and in Vivo; Mechanism for Anti-Thyroid Activity of Soy," presented at the November 1999 Soy Symposium in Washington, DC, National Center for Toxicological Research, Jefferson, AR.

50. Brian Ross and Richard D. Allyn, "The Other Side of Soy," June 9, 2000. **http://web.archive.org/web/20000815204236/ http://abcnews.go.com/onair/2020/2020_000609_soy_ feature.html**

51. Ibid.

52. Dr. Joseph Mercola, "Soy is an Endocrine Disrupter and Can Disrupt Your Child's Health." (January 16, 2002). **www.mercola.com**

53. C. Irvine, M. Fitzpatrick, I. Robertson, D. Woodhams, et al., "The Potential Adverse Effects of Soybean Phytoestrogens in Infant Feeding," *New Zealand Medical Journal* (May 24, 1995): 318.

54. K. B. Delclos, T. J. Bucci, et al., "Effects of Dietary Genistein Exposure During Development on Male and Female CD (Sprague-Dawley) Rats," *Reproductive Toxicology* 15, no. 6 (2001): 647–663; W. N. Jefferson, J. F. Couse, E. Padilla-Banks, et al., "Neonatal Exposure to Genistein Induces Estrogen Receptor (ER) Alpha Expression and Multioocyte Follicles in the Maturing Mouse Ovary: Evidence for ERbeta-mediated and Nonestrogenic Actions," *Biology of Reproduction* 67, no. 4 (2002): 1285–1296; W. N. Jefferson, E. Padilla-Banks and R. Newbold, "Adverse Effects on Female Development and Reproduction in CD-1 Mice Following Neonatal Exposure to the Phytoestrogen Genistein at Environmentally Relevant Doses," *Biology of Reproduction* 73, no. 4 (2005): 798–806; W. N. Jefferson, R. Newbold, E. Padilla-Banks and M. Pepling, "Neonatal Genistein

Treatment Alters Ovarian Differentiation in the Mouse: Inhibition of Oocyte Nest Breakdown and Increased Oocyte Survival," *Biology of Reproduction* 74, no. 1 (2006):161–168; T. Kouki, M. Kishitake, et al., "Effects of Neonatal Treatment with Phytoestrogens, Genistein and Daidzein on Sex Difference in Female Rat Brain Function: Estrous Cycle and Lordosis," *Hormones and Behavior* 44, no. 2 (2003): 140–145; T. Nagao, S. Yoshimura, et al., "Reproductive Effects in Male and Female Rats of Neonatal Exposure to Genistein," *Reproductive Toxicology* 15, no. 4 (2001): 399–411; Y. Nikaido, K. Yoshizawa, et al, "Effects of Maternal Xenoestrogen Exposure on Development of the Reproductive Tract and Mammary Gland in Female CD-1 Mouse Offspring," *Reproductive Toxicology* 18, no. 6 (2004):803–811; P. L. Whitten, C. Lewis, et al., "A Phytoestrogen Diet Induces the Premature Anovulatory Syndrome in Lactationally Exposed Female Rats," *Biology of Reproduction* 49, no. 5 (1993): 1117–1121.

55. T. C. Campbell and J. Chen, "Diet and Chronic Degenerative Diseases" in *Western Diseases: Their Dietary Prevention and Reversibility.* Edited by N. J. Temple and D. P. Burkitt (Totowa, N.J.: Humana Press, 1994): 67–119.

56. National Center for Health Statistics Data Brief Number 49, November 2010. Trends in Intake of Energy and Macrontrients in Adults from 1999–2000 through 2007–2008; Jacqueline D. Wright, Dr. P.H., and Chia-Yih Wang, Ph.D. From the website of the Centers for Disease Control and Prevention. www.cdc.gov/nchs/data/databriefs/db49.htm

57. Dr. Norman Walker, *Become Younger* (Summertown, TN: Norwalk Press, 1995), 63.

58. Brian Shilhavy and Marianita Shilhavy, *Virgin Coconut Oil* (West Bend, WI: Tropical Traditions, Inc., 2004).

59. A general review of citations for problems with polyunsaturate consumption is found in Edward R. Pinckney, M.D. and Cathey Pinckney, *The Cholesterol Controversy* (Los Angeles: Sherbourne Press, 1973), 127–131. Research indicating the correlation of polyunsaturates with learning problems is found in D. Harmon, et al., *Journal of the American Geriatrics Society*, 24, no. 1 (1976): 292–298; Z. Meerson, et al., *Bull Exp Bio Med* 96, no. 9 (1983): 70–71. Regarding weight gain, levels of linoleic acid in adipose tissues reflect the amount of linoleic acid in the diet, see Valero, et al., *Annals of Nutrition and Metabolism* 34, no. 6 (November–December 1990): 323–327; C. V. Felton, et al. *Lancet* 344 (1994): 1195–1196.

60. Peter Jaret, "Understanding the Omega Fatty Acids." www.webmd.com/diet/healthy-kitchen-11/omega-fatty-acids?page=2

61. Ibid.

62. Dr. Gary Farr, "Comparing Organic Versus Commercially Grown Foods," Rutgers University Study, New Brunswick, NJ, 2002.

63. Dr. Edward Howell, *Enzyme Nutrition: The Food Enzyme Concept.* (New York: Avery, 1995), 31–32. Howell refers to Dr. Troland's quote as coming from a paper he wrote in 1916 titled "The Enzyme Theory of Life," for a medical journal.

64. Ibid., xv.

65. Tom Bohager, *Enzymes: What the Experts Know* (Prescott, AZ: One World Press, 2006), 10.

66. Howell, *Enzyme Nutrition,* 27.

CHAPTER FOUR

1. Shinya, *The Enzyme Factor.*

2. Chris Gaugler, "Lipofuscin," *Stanislaus Journal of Biochemical Reviews* (May 1997).

3. I. A. Prior, F. Davidson, C. E. Salmond and Z. Czochanska, "Cholesterol, Coconuts and Diet on Polynesian Atolls: A Natural Experiment: The Pukapuka and Tokelau Island Studies," *American Journal of Clinical Nutrition* 34, no. 8 (1981).

4. B. Hornung, E. Amtmann and G. Sauer, "Lauric Acid Inhibits the Maturation of Vesicular Stomatitis Virus," *Journal of General Virology* 75 (1994); H. Kaunitz, "Medium-chain Triglycerides (MCT) in Aging and Arteriosclerosis," *Journal of Environmental Pathology, Toxicology, and Oncology* 6, nos. 3–4 (1986); H. Kaunitz and C. S. Dayrit, "Coconut Oil Consumption and Coronary Heart Disease," *Philippine Journal of Internal Medicine* (1992): 30; P. A. Kurup and T. Rajmohan, "Consumption of Coconut Oil and Coconut Kernal and the Incidence of Atherosclerosis," in *Coconut and Coconut Oil in Human Nutrition, Proceedings,* symposium on Coconut and Coconut Oil in Human Nutrition, sponsored by the Coconut Development Board, Kochi, India, March 27, 1994.

5. Haas, *Staying Healthy with Nutrition*, 49.

6. W. C. Grant, "Influence of Avocados on Serum Cholesterol," *Proceedings of the Society for Experimental Biology and Medicine* 104 (1960): 45–47.

7. Sir Stanley Davidson, R. Passmore and M. A. Eastwood, *Human Nutrition and Dietics* (Philadelphia: Churchill Livingston, 1986).

8. Cousens, *Conscious Eating*, 474.

9. N. W. Walker, D.Sc., *Fresh Vegetable and Fruit Juices* (Norwalk Press: Summertown, TN, 1978), 57.

10. Professor Arnold Ehret. *Mucusless Diet Healing System: A Scientific Method of Eating Your Way to Health.* (New York: Benedict Lust Publications, 2002), 79.

11. H. R. Maurer, "Bromelain: Biochemistry, Pharmacology and Medical Use." *Cellular and Molecular Life Sciences* 58; no. 9 (August 2001): 1243–1245.

12. www.herbs2000.com/herbs/herbs_pineapple.htm

13. S. Helms, A. Miller, "Natural Treatment of Chronic Rhinosinusitis." *Alternative Medicine Review* 3 (September 2011): 190–207.

14. Cathy Wong, "Bromelain." About.com Guide. October 3, 2011. http://altmedicine.about.com/cs/herbsvitaminsa1/a/Bromelain.htm

15. Johnson, *The Sugar Fix*, 199.

16. Pineapple. Review of Natural Products. Facts & Comparisons 4.0 (St. Louis, MO: Wolters Kluwer Health, Inc., January 2009).

17. Peter T. Pugliese, M.D., "Vitamin E: A Skin Care Ally," *Skin, Inc. Magazine* (September 2009). www.skininc.com/skinscience/ingredients/55400207.html?page=4

18. Catherine Boal, "Antioxidant-Rich Almonds on a Par with Fruits and Vegetables" (June 26, 2008). www.nutraingredients.com/Research/Antioxidant-rich-almonds-on-a-par-with-fruit-and-vegetables

19. Rosalie K. Woods, E. Haydn Walters, Joan M. Raven, Rory Wolfe, "Food and Nutrient Intakes and Asthma Risk in Young Adults." *American Journal of Clinical Nutrition* 78, no. 3 (September 2003): 414–421.

20. Shinya, *The Enzyme Factor*, 100.

21. E. Isolauri, "Probiotics: From Anecdotes to Clinical Demonstration," *Journal of Allergy and Clinical Immunology* 100, no. 6 (December 2001): 1062; H. Majamaa and E. Isolauri, "Probiotics: A Novel Approach in the Management of Food Allergy," *Journal of Allergy and Clinical Immunology* 99, no. 2 (February 1997): 179–185; R. D. Rolfe, "The Role of Probiotic Cultures in the Control of Gastrointestinal Health," *Journal of Nutrition,* 130, Supplement 2S (February 2000): 396S–402S; J. M. Saavedra and A. Tschernia, "Human Studies with Probiotics and Prebiotics: Clinical Implications," *British Journal of Nutrition* 87, Supplement 2 (May 2002): S241–S246.

22. Shinya, *The Enzyme Factor,* 121.

23. Phyllis A. Balch, C.N.C., *Prescription for Nutritional Healing* (New York: Avery Books, 2000), 23.

24. Parris M. Kidd, Ph.D., "Glutathione: Systemic Protectant Against Oxidative and Free Radical Damage," *Alternative Medicine Review* 2, no. 3 (2001): 161–165.

25. M. Keophiphath, F. Priem, I. Jacquemond-Oullet, et al., "Vinyldithiin from Garlic Inhibits Differentiation and Inflammation of Human Preadipocytes," *Journal of Nutrition* 139, no. 11 (November 2009): 2055–2060; S. Mukherjee, I. Lekli, S. Goswami, et al., "Freshly Crushed Garlic Is a Superior Cardioprotective Agent Than Processed

Garlic," *Journal of Agriculture and Food Chemistry* 57, no. 15 (August 12, 2009): 7137–7144; K. Ried, O. R. Frank, N. P. Stocks, et al., "Effect of Garlic on Blood Pressure: A Systematic Review and Meta-analysis," *BMC Cardiovascular Disorders* 8, no. 13 (June 16, 2008); G. Siegel, F. Michel, M. Ploch, M. Rodriguez, et al., "Inhibition of Arteriosclerotic Plaque Development by Garlic," *Wien Med Wochenschr* (2004).

CHAPTER FIVE

1. Ehret, *Mucusless Diet Healing System*, 79.

CHAPTER SIX

1. Viktoras Kulvinskas, *Survival into the 21st Century* (Wethersfield, CT: Omangod Press, 1975), 197.

2. Elisabeth Bergman, "Beet Juice Lowers Blood Pressure: Nitrates Found in Vegetables May Protect Blood Vessels," referencing A. Webb, *Hypertension* (February 4, 2008). **www.webmd.com/ hypertension-high-blood-pressure/news/20080208/ beet-juice-lowers-blood-pressure**

3. P. Knekt, S. Isotupa, H. Rissanen, et al., "Quercetin Intake and the Incidence of Cerebrovascular Disease," *European Journal of Clinical Nutrition* 54 (2000): 415–417.

4. Jeanelle Boyer and Rui H. Liu. "Apple Phytochemicals and Their Health Benefits," *Nutrition Journal* 3, no. 5 (May 12, 2004) doi:10.118611475-2891-3-5. **www.nutritionnj.com/content/3/1/5**

CHAPTER SEVEN

1. C. Hoelzl, H. Glatt, T. Simic, et al., "DNA Protective Effects of Brussels Sprouts: Results of a Human Intervention Study," *AACR Meeting Abstracts* (December 2007): B67. **www.whfoods.com/genpage. php?tname=foodspice&dbid=10**

2. P. Brat, S. George, A. Bellamy, et al., "Daily Polyphenol Intake in France from Fruit and Vegetables," *Journal of Nutrition* 136 (September 2006): 2368–2573.

3. A. Rawlings, "Cellulite and Its Treatment," *International Journal of Cosmetic Science* 28 (2006): 175–190.

4. Dr. David Williams, *Alternative (For the Health Conscious Individual)* 7, no. 12 (June 1998).

5. Y. Omura, Y. Shimotsuura, A. Fukuoka, et al. "Significant Mercury Deposits in Internal Organs Following the Removal of Dental Amalgam, Development of Pre-Cancer on the Gingiva and the Sides of the Tongue and Their Represented Organs as a Result of Inadvertent Exposure to Strong Curing Light (Used to Solidify Synthetic Dental Filling Material), Effective Treatment: A Clinical Case Report, Along with Organ Representation Areas for Each Tooth"; *Acupunct Electrother Res* 21, no. 2 (April–June 1996): 133–160.

6. Excerpt from a lecture, *The Klinghardt Neurotoxin Elimination Protocol,* presented by Dietrich Klinghardt, M.D., Ph.D., at the Jean Piaget Department at the University of Geneva, Switzerland, October 2002 to physicians and dentists from Europe, Israel, several Arab countries and Asia. Approved by: American Academy of Neural Therapy and Institute of Neurobiology (Bellevue, WA, USA), Institute for Neurobiologie (Stuttgart, Germany), Academy for Balanced NeuroBiology Ltd. (London, United Kingdom).

7. Ibid.

8. Haas and Levin, *Staying Healthy with Nutrition,* 609, 766.

9. M. K. Jensen, P. Koh-Banerjee, F. B. Hu, M. Franz, et al., "Intakes of Whole Grains, Bran, and Germ and the Risk of Coronary Heart Disease in Men." *American Journal of Clinical Nutrition* 80, no. 6 (December 2004):1492–1499. PMID: 15585760.

10. P. Koh-Banerjee, M. Franz, L. Sampson, et al. "Changes in whole-grain, bran, and cereal fiber consumption in relation to 8-y weight gain among men." *American Journal of Clinical Nutrition* 80, no. 5 (November 2004):1237–1245. PMID: 15531671.

11. L. Liu, L. Zubik, F. W. Collins, et al. "The Antiatherogenic Potential of Oat Phenolic Compounds." *Atherosclerosis* 175, no. 1 (July 2004):39–49. PMID: 15186945.

12. L. Nie, M. L. Wise, D. M. Peterson, et al. "Avenanthramide, a Polyphenol from Oats, Inhibits Vascular Smooth Muscle Cell Proliferation and Enhances Nitric Oxide Production," *Atherosclerosis* 186, no. 2 (June 2006):260–266. PMID: 16139284.

CHAPTER EIGHT

1. Cousens, *Conscious Eating,* 612.

2. Ibid., 611.

3. Gary Null, Ph.D., *The Complete Encyclopedia of Natural Healing: A Comprehensive A–Z Listing of Common and Chronic Illnesses and their Proven Treatments*. (New York: Kensington Publishing Corp., 2005).

4. www.ncbi.nlm.nih.gov/pubmed/10921251

5. Ethan A. Huff, "Discover the Radiation Protective Benefits of Spirulina and Chlorella," *Natural News* (March 21, 2011). www.naturalnews.com/031779_spirulina_radiation. html#ixzz1aKxjtQx6

6. Toru Mizoguchi, Isao Takehara, Tohru Masuzawa, et al., "Nutrigenomic Studies of Effects of Chlorella on Subjects with High-Risk Factors for Lifestyle-Related Disease," *Journal of Medicinal Food* 3 (September 11, 2008): 395–404.

CHAPTER ELEVEN

1. A. Goodson, W. Summerfield and I. Cooper, "Survey of Bisphenol A and Bisphenol F in Canned Foods," *Food Additive Contamination* 19 (2002):796–802. www.ewg.org/node/20941

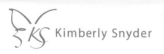
Kimberly Snyder

GET FREE ACCESS TO
KIMBERLY SNYDER'S
BEAUTY DETOX COMMUNITY

THE **BEAUTY DETOX** MOVEMENT
HAS SPREAD TO OVER

150 COUNTRIES WORLDWIDE

Join Hundreds Of Thousands
of like-minded individuals all interested in creating a
new healthy lifestyle like you.

People within our community enjoy free access to Kimberly's recipes,
weight loss advice, beauty tips, and product recommendations.

Simply Go To
www.KimberlySnyder.net
& Sign Up Now To Get Instant Access

It's 100% Free!

INDEX

ABOUT THE AUTHOR

Kimberly Snyder, C.N., is a celebrity nutritionist and bestselling author of *The Beauty Detox Solution.*

Snyder is the go-to nutritionist for many of the entertainment industry's top celebrities. She has worked with and/or prepared food for Drew Barrymore, Fergie, Hilary Duff, Dita Von Teese, Rooney Mara, Kate Mara, Kerry Washington, LeAnn Rimes, Channing Tatum, Josh Duhamel, Vince Vaughn, Owen Wilson, Ben Stiller, Christine Taylor, Kevin James, Chris Hemsworth, Leslie Mann, Olivia Wilde, Jimmy Fallon, Jason Bateman, Melissa McCarthy, Kristen Bell, Malin Akerman, Laura Benanti, Tom Hiddleston, Eddie Cibrian, Justin Long, Mark Ruffalo and many others. Snyder has also prepared food on film sets such as *The Avengers, 21 Jump Street, Transformers 3, The Internship, The Secret Life of Walter Mitty, The Watch, Couples Retreat, Going the Distance, The Dilemma* and *Hall Pass.*

Snyder is also a recurring nutritional and beauty expert on the *Today* show, *The Dr. Oz Show* and *Good Day LA* and has also been featured on *Good Morning America, Access Hollywood Live, EXTRA, E! Entertainment, Fox & Friends* and *Better TV.* She has also been profiled in the *New York Times* as well as top national magazines including *Vogue, Harper's Bazaar, InStyle, USA TODAY, Lucky, Elle, Marie Claire, Redbook, Allure, Esquire, Prevention, Shape, Health, Details, Nylon, Whole Living, Fitness, People, People StyleWatch, Us Weekly* and *Parade* magazine among many others.

After graduating magna cum laude from Georgetown University, Snyder didn't choose an ordinary path. Instead, she embarked on a three-year solo journey spanning over fifty countries and six continents, exposing her to a wide range of health and beauty modalities and approaches from different cultures.

Snyder is a member of the National Association of Nutrition Professionals and the American Association of Nutrition Consultants, and is the founder of Kimberly Snyder's GLOW BIO, a 100% organic smoothie and juice emporium in West Hollywood. Snyder is also the founder of The Glowing Lean System.® Her health and beauty blog at www.KimberlySnyder.net has spawned the Beauty Detox movement, a worldwide community that includes members in over 150 countries.